"What an inspiration to read Jenni's amazing story about recovering from an eating disorder and falling in love with herself and life. Writing from the heart with sincerity and wisdom, she provides insight, hope, and motivation for those in a battle with their body and self. This uplifting book is a must read for anyone with an eating disorder or who cares about someone who suffers from anorexia nervosa or bulimia."

—*Ann Kearney-Cooke, Ph.D.; Distinguished Scholar, Partnership for Gender-Specific Medicine, Columbia University; and author of* Change Your Mind, Change Your Body: Feeling Good About Your Body and Self After 40

"This book is exactly what the eating disorders community needs. *Good-Bye Ed, Hello Me* breaks the chains of the 'recovery' journey and embarks on a whole new frontier—real life. Jenni's signature wit, sense of humor, and authenticity help readers—whether they are parents, patients, or professionals—get past looking at the disease and turn the focus to what matters: the person. Providing enduring hope and inspiring her readers to action, Jenni has done it again!"

—*Kirsten Haglund, Miss America 2008*

"In *Good-Bye Ed, Hello Me*, Jenni gives us a stunning personal account of what life can be when you truly, really, completely recover from an eating disorder. She promises 'full freedom' and assures us that a life filled with love, laughter, and true happiness is waiting. Thank you, Jenni, for sharing your journey and telling all those who suffer from eating disorders, 'yes, you can!'"

—*Kitty Westin, M.A., LP; President, Eating Disorders Coalition for Research, Policy & Action*

"Jenni's compassionate follow-up to *Life Without Ed* provides inspiration to every person struggling with an eating disorder. Her candid memoir gives hope to the hopeless, beyond beating an eating disorder. Life gets ever so much better—told by someone who has battled the body bashing, eating wars, and mind games to emerge wiser, joyous, and authentic. Good-bye, eating disorder; hello, thriving life!"

—Evelyn Tribole, M.S., RD;
coauthor of Intuitive Eating

"Jenni Schaefer's *Good-Bye Ed, Hello Me* is a powerful answer to the question many sufferers of ED ask: What will my life look like when it's not controlled by Ed? By highlighting her own struggle along the way to her recovery, Schaefer demonstrates there is hope for everyone who chooses to start along the path. As she rightly notes, 'with recovery, anything is possible!'"

—Jess Weiner, author of A Very Hungry Girl *and*
Life Doesn't Begin 5 Pounds from Now

"Readers not only will learn how to fall in love with life but also will fall in love with Jenni Schaefer's second book, *Good-Bye, Ed, Hello Me.* Jenni has beautifully crafted a tale of her journey into wellness that is at once practical, poetic, and promising. Both clinicians and clients alike can benefit from this inside look at what it takes on a body/mind level to fully recover from the tenacious grip of an eating disorder. Especially helpful are Jenni's focus on body image, the steps necessary to take in order to shift away from the disease identity, and how to overcome feeling 'weird' when you are actually feeling 'good.'"

—Adrienne Ressler, LMSW, CEDS;
National Training Director,
the Renfrew Center Foundation

goodbye ed, hello me

Recover from Your *Eating Disorder* and Fall in Love with Life

Jenni Schaefer

New York   Chicago   San Francisco   Lisbon   London   Madrid   Mexico City
Milan   New Delhi   San Juan   Seoul   Singapore   Sydney   Toronto

The McGraw-Hill Companies

Library of Congress Cataloging-in-Publication Data

Schaefer, Jenni.
  Good-bye Ed, hello me : recover from your eating disorder and fall in love with life / Jenni Schaefer.
      p.   cm.
  ISBN 978-0-07-160887-9 (alk. paper)
  1. Schaefer, Jenni—Health.   2. Eating disorders—Patients—
Biography.   3. Eating disorders—Treatment—Case studies.   I. Title.

  RC552.E18S344   2010
  362.196'85260092—dc22   2009008596

    6 7 8 9 10 11 12 13 14 15 16 17 18 19 20 21 22 QFR/QFR 1 5 4 3 2

ISBN 978-0-07-160887-9
MHID   0-07-160887-7

McGraw-Hill books are available at special quantity discou nts to use as premiums and sales promotions or for use in corporate training programs. To contact a representative, please e-mail us at bulksales@mcgraw-hill.com.

This book provides a variety of ideas and suggestions. It is sold with the understanding that the publisher and author are not rendering psychological, medical, or professional services. The author is not a doctor or psychologist, and the information in this book is the author's own opinion, unless otherwise stated. The information contained in this book is intended to provide helpful and informative material on eating disorders. It is not intended to serve as a replacement for professional medical or psychological advice. All medical, dietetic, or therapeutic recommendations mentioned in this book are not meant to be taken without the advice of a medical doctor, registered dietician, and/or licensed therapist.

The names of many of the people mentioned in this book have been changed, as have certain physical characteristics and other descriptive details. Some of the events and characters are also composites of several individual events or persons.

This book is printed on acid-free paper.

To my fellow Ed-busters,

those recovering from eating disorders, those who are

recovered, family members and friends, and all of the

professionals working tirelessly for hope and healing

Contents

3

The Dating Game: *Exploring the World* — 73

4

Getting Engaged: *Relationships and More* — 101

5

The White Dress:
A Healthy Body and Positive Body Image — 129

6

The Perfectly Imperfect Wedding:
Overcoming Perfectionism — 163

7

Happily Married: *Falling in Love with Life* — 193

* *denotes chapters with exercises*

Foreword

I RECOVERED FROM my own eating disorder long before Jenni Schaefer was born. But now she and I are on the same team, helping others overcome this devastating illness.

Jenni has truly won her battle with her eating disorder, and she carries the wisdom, grace, energy, and enthusiasm necessary to inspire others to do the same. As hard as it is to believe, when I first recovered there were still no books available on the topic. I was a lone figure not just because I had suffered from an illness most people did not know existed, but even more so because I had recovered and become a therapist treating others to make a full recovery too.

Over the years I would continue to hear—not only from my patients but from sufferers out in the world—that seeing someone who had recovered was important, even crucial, to their belief in their own ability to leave their eating disorders behind and get well. Some professionals told me to be careful about identifying myself too much with being recovered. One leader in the field asked, "Do you want to be known as being a recovered anorexic or as being a good therapist?" I went away worried. But soon after I made a decision that I could be both. And I am.

Being a source of hope and a role model of recovery has been part of my mission over the years. Jenni has taken that mission to new depths and heights. Through her writing, her singing, her workshops, and her example of a life fully lived, she is a source of healing in a still-crazy world.

Since you are holding this book, you too must be interested in a better life, free from the trappings of an eating disorder. This book is about being really free. What you will find on these pages is a guide to recovering fully, but even more, to finding joy and peace in your life. This book is a journey through Jenni's process of connecting back to herself and to living a complete life. Sharing her process will help many of you do the same. You will also benefit from the pearls of wisdom Jenni has received from many of her mentors and leaders in the field of eating disorders, such as Craig Johnson, Cynthia Bulik, Ovidio Bermudez, and Evelyn Tribole, as well as from feminist soul sisters such as Anita Johnston and Margo Maine. Jenni has done her work and her homework and passes it on with every page.

When I first met Jenni, she was still identifying herself as being "in recovery." I asked her why, explaining that the term is so broad I wonder exactly what it means to each person who uses it. I also was worried about her message regarding "Ed" in that I had seen clients use the metaphor as an excuse for their behavior—"Ed made me do it." True to the person she is, Jenni has looked at both of these issues over the last few years and gone far beyond them in *Good-Bye Ed, Hello Me.*

In this book, Jenni discusses how appropriate it is for her to call herself "recovered" and what that means to her, but in her non-judgmental way, she leaves room for you to find what term best suits your situation. Instead of telling you how to deal with Ed, this book explains how to let go of the past, deal with the present, love your body, and live your authentic life. Passing on learned wisdom, Jenni says, "We can't give away what we don't have," and you will find that she "has it." From sharing how she handles her perfectionism to dealing with a jar of thigh cream, she not only takes you through her personal experiences but helps direct you in how to make it your own. She makes recovery and full living seem possible for everyone, although she is clear that it is not easy: "Fully recovering from my eating disorder felt just like someone had asked me to become left-handed." She is right. I always ask my clients to share with me and their loved ones the answer to the question, "Why does getting better feel so bad?" Their replies not only help others understand how hard it is to get better but lead to a better understanding of what might be keeping someone stuck.

This book is about getting out of the stuck places. I suspect you will laugh and cry. You will find yourself somewhere on these pages, and you will also find hope that things can be better. Toward the end of the book, Jenni says, "Real hope combined with real action has always pulled me through difficult times. Real hope combined with doing nothing has never pulled me through." I find it a matter of great synchronicity that I read these words right after President Obama's incredibly hopeful inauguration speech. Jenni has timed it just right. People of all persuasions in all situations and circumstances need hope, but they also need help in combining that hope with action. *Good-Bye Ed, Hello Me* is a book to help those with eating disorders do just that.

CAROLYN COSTIN, LMFT, M.A., M.ED.
Director, Monte Nido Treatment Center & Affiliates
Author of *The Eating Disorder Sourcebook, Your Dieting
    Daughter,* and *100 Questions and Answers About
    Eating Disorders*
www.montenido.com

Acknowledgments

FOLLOWING THIS BOOK'S guidance on perfectionism, I am not going to try to write this anywhere near perfectly. I could actually write an entire book just acknowledging all of the people who have helped me along the way. You know who you are: *thank you from the bottom of my heart.*

To my amazing family, in sharing my story, I am also sharing yours. Thank you for your support in that. I am deeply grateful for my parents, Joe and Susan Schaefer. I could not ask for a better mom and dad. To my older brother, Steven Schaefer, and his wife, Destiny, thank you for always being there with love and laughter. Much of that laughter has been inspired by your two children, my adorable nephews, Andrew and Aiden. To my younger brother, Jeffery Schaefer, thank you for just being you—for always responding to my e-mails, texts, and calls about this book and life in general.

You would not be holding this book without four incredibly talented people in publishing. To my editor, John Aherne, thanks for your great insight and your boundless energy for this project. To my literary agent, Linda Loewenthal, thanks for wholeheartedly believing in this book from day one. And to Sarah Pelz and Ann Pryor, I appreciate your enthusiasm and expertise regarding both *Good-Bye Ed, Hello Me* and *Life Without Ed.*

Thanks to all of you who read *Life Without Ed.* Your support of that book made it possible for me to write this one. And to all of the health care professionals who guided me to finding not only a life without Ed but also one with joy, love, and peace, thank you. I especially want to recognize Trish Sanders, LPC/MHSP, for helping me find my voice.

I send out a big thanks to the wonderful professionals in all of the recovery fields who have embraced my work from the very beginning. I want to acknowledge those who took time out of their busy schedules to review various parts of this book to ensure its accuracy: Ovidio Bermudez, M.D.; Michael E. Berrett, Ph.D.; Cynthia Bulik, Ph.D., FAED; Carolyn Costin, LMFT, M.A., M.Ed. (Thanks also for writing such a wonderful foreword, Carolyn!); Craig Johnson, Ph.D.; Anita Johnston, Ph.D.; Walter Kaye, M.D.; Margo Maine, Ph.D.; Kimberly Passmore, RD, CD; Adrienne Ressler, LMSW; and Evelyn Tribole, M.S., RD. Thanks to all of you, this book is that much better!

To Lynn Grefe, I appreciate your reading of the entire manuscript and the important insight you provided at the very end of the writing process; it made a big difference. Thanks to Mark Schwartz, Sc.D., who specifically inspired the section titled "Getting to Know Ed." To Sondra Kronberg, M.S., RD, CDN, I will never forget you as the first person who believed in me enough to fly me out of town to present to your group. You started it all!

Thank you to my friends. I wish I could mention all of you, but that would be a little perfectionistic of me. To Dave Berg and Georgia Middleman, who are not only incredible friends but incredible singer-songwriters as well, thank you for helping to make the song in the back of this book possible. Thanks to Melanie Aldis, Sandi Everett, Melody Robinson, and Aaron Sparkman for being great friends and for allowing me to share a bit about you on these pages. To the Whitman family (Rich, Debra, Chris, Nick, and Nicole) in Kerrville, Texas, your love and encouragement (and all the motorcycle rides) have meant more to me than you can imagine. Thank you to Rob Simbeck for reading the manuscript and helping me so much over the years to get the word out about my work. And to William McInnes, your support has made it possible for me to share my hope with individuals—one by one—across the globe.

A special thanks to Dr. Phil McGraw and his staff both for supporting my work and for your efforts in getting the word out about eating disorders.

To those touched by eating disorders, you inspire me to keep moving forward in my work and life. Thanks to you, this book is about life!

Last but definitely not least, I thank God for my many blessings.

Introduction

I SKIPPED MY FIRST marriage. The wedding invitations were stamped but not mailed, and three pink bridesmaid dresses were bought but never worn. My beautiful wedding gown was sold at a consignment store in Dallas before I even had a chance to wear it, and the matching white satin shoes are shoved somewhere in the back of my closet.

My wedding day—August 6, 2005—came and went, and I was still single. As I was about to join hands with Mark, my husband-to-be, and begin our life together, I let go, turned around, and walked away. I was not going to walk down the aisle at my big Texas wedding and make a huge mistake. My husband-to-be was not-to-be for me.

Since the wedding—and marriage—did *not* take off as planned (major understatement), people in my life worried that my ex from years past would show up to provide comfort and support. They thought for sure that Ed would sneak back into my life.

Ed and I did not get back together. In fact, the possibility did not even cross my mind. The last thing I needed during that difficult time was to bring something even more difficult into my life. It took a long time to call it quits with Ed, and I won't go back.

You might know that Ed stands for *eating disorder* (the acronym ED). I learned in therapy to treat my eating disorder like a relationship rather than an illness or a condition. I learned to think of it as a distinct being with unique thoughts and a personality separate from my own. In recovery, I continually practiced separating Ed's voice from mine. I learned that Ed—not Jenni—was the one saying, "You're fat," "Don't eat that," and "You're not good enough." Throughout recovery, I separated from Ed and made room for the real, authentic Jenni to exist. Ed was very much like an abusive husband, so sometimes I say that I divorced Ed.

I did not rebound to Ed even though breaking up with Mark and the circumstances surrounding it were excruciatingly painful. While Mark and I had several issues that needed work (as most relationships do), the one that propelled me to give back the ring was alcohol. I could not marry a man who, from my point of view, often drank so much at night that he didn't remember conversations the next day. I felt like he loved alcohol more than me. From my experience in recovery, I knew that wasn't true. At least, my head knew it—my heart never did.

All in all, at the end of day on August 6, 2005, I was not married—not to Mark *and* not to Ed. I am fully recovered.

When I was in the process of writing my first book, *Life Without Ed*, I considered myself to be "significantly recovered" from my eating disorder. I was doing well in recovery—relatively free from eating disordered behaviors—but I still talked to Ed a lot. As I write this book, I am "fully recovered." I'm free from eating disordered behaviors, and I don't talk to Ed anymore. (Yes, it gets this good!) To get to this point, I devoted many more years to being "in recovery."

Good-Bye Ed, Hello Me is the difference (and it is a big one) between being in recovery and being fully recovered. To me, the latter means both breaking free from destructive behaviors with food and having a healthy relationship with my body, as well as finding joy and peace in my life. I can't pinpoint when this shift happened for me, but what I can say for sure is that after making the leap to fully recovered, it became important for me to claim it.

I specifically asked my friend and colleague Carolyn Costin, LMFT, M.A., M.Ed., to write the foreword to this book, because she is the first person who truly encouraged me to claim myself as fully recovered. Thanks to her wisdom, my outlook on life—both personally and professionally—has changed for the better. As long as I kept referring to myself as being in recovery from my eating disorder, I was giving Ed a place in my life. This was a self-fulfilling prophecy for me: as long as I believed Ed would haunt me, he did. So I stopped believing it.

It is important to note that I did not let my guard down in the beginning. In other words, during the first moments that I believed I was fully recovered, I established a perimeter of caution. This does not mean that I lived in constant terror of Ed returning, but it means that I stayed the course with therapy and kept one eye open for him—just in case he was lurking around, trying to catch me in a moment of overconfidence.

I began accepting and claiming the state of fully recovered for myself after I had made it through many difficult times over a period of several years without turning to Ed. Some true tests for me were dealing with my broken engagement, my dad's diagnosis of cancer, and a friend's death. Not once during these challenging times did I go back to Ed. I didn't even think about it. I no longer use the metaphor of Ed in my everyday life at all. I only speak the language of Ed in my work as an educator.

If you've read *Life Without Ed*, you know that during recovery from my eating disorder, I learned to personify the voice of my perfectionism as Ms. Perfectionist. When I was still speaking in terms of Ed and trying to separate from him, Ms. Perfectionist was a helpful tool to let me separate from perfectionism as well. But after I developed a healthy relationship with food and stopped using the metaphor of Ed, the metaphor of Ms. Perfectionist fell away as well—unfortunately, the perfectionism stayed with me full force. (Without Ed for relief, I had no idea how to deal with perfectionism, so it seemed stronger than ever.) At this point, I began thinking of it in more global terms. So in this book, you will not read specifically about Ms. Perfectionist, but you will read a lot about perfectionism. In fact, dealing with my perfectionistic tendencies has been so important in my life that I've dedicated Part 6 of this book to it. If it helps for you to name your perfectionism, by all means, do it. We all must find what works for us.

Part 5 of this book is dedicated to learning how to love, nurture, and respect your body. Years ago (prerecovery), I would have read some of the sections about body image and thought, "Yeah, right. I'll never be able to love my new, healthy body. Impossible." Since I wouldn't have even believed myself, I realize that you might have a difficult time believing me, so I'm warning you up front: this is just how recovered you can be! Are you ready?

Negative body image seems to be one of Ed's last-ditch efforts to keep us under his control. If he can keep us hating our bodies (even long after our eating disorder behaviors subside), then he still holds the power to work himself back into our lives. Negative body image was the last aspect of my eating disorder to go, but it *did* go. This makes sense to me, since it was the first to come along.

When I was only a four-year-old in dance class, Ed whispered in my ear that I was fat. His voice grew louder as I grew older. He encouraged me to restrict food, which then led to bingeing and purging. When I entered college and was living away from home for the first time, I slid down fast into anorexia and bulimia.

I even turned down an acceptance to medical school after graduation, because I knew that my eating behaviors combined with perfectionism would kill me in such a competitive environment. Instead of beginning the path to become a doctor, I moved to Nashville (Music City, USA) to sing. It turns out that the competition there was just as fierce as it would have been in medical school, only I was singing instead of studying. Needless to say, I hit rock bottom with Ed and finally made a decision to get professional help. With lots of time and patience, I recovered.

Throughout this book, you will see the words *time* and *patience* a lot. So much of recovery is just that. When we talk about recovering from eating disorders, we are talking about years, not months.

Another word you will see a lot is *pain*. I have heard people in recovery from alcoholism say, "Pain before sobriety and pain before serenity." I have found this quote to be accurate for eating disorders as well. Intense pain often pushed me to make changes. The pain of the eating disorder pushed me into recovering from eating-disordered behaviors, and then the emotional turmoil I experienced without those behaviors (not knowing how to cope with perfectionism, feelings, and life in general) took me even further, so that I ultimately found serenity. I'm not sure if I would ever have reached this point in my life had it not been for my eating disorder. Ed pushed me to become a healthier person than I probably would have been without him. I would never go back and choose to have an eating disorder (it was *that* painful), but I am deeply grateful for the gifts of recovery.

In this book, it might sometimes seem like recovery was simple for me, because no amount of words can adequately explain the struggle of overcoming an eating disorder. Trust me when I say that recovering from mine was the most difficult thing I have ever done in my life. I actually never thought I would fully recover, but I did.

Now I have the privilege of sharing my story with you as a writer and speaker. I still live in Nashville and am excited that I have the opportunity to incorporate music into my work as well. If you check out the new song in the back of this book, you will notice that it is not specifically about eating disorders. Now that I am fully recovered, I'm in a position to write and sing about anything at all. Don't be surprised if my next book is about dating or music or possibly even fiction. As you move further away from Ed and more toward life, you too will discover that the possibilities are endless!

Since Ed and I don't talk these days, *Good-Bye Ed, Hello Me* is more about life than it is about Ed. You already know how horrible Ed can be, but you might not know how wonderful life can be. And you might not know Jenni, the woman behind the eating disorder. As I tell you about my journey, I want you to get to know me.

On my journey, spirituality was important. Even though I will share some of what I have learned, I welcome the fact that everyone has different beliefs and even more different paths to finding those beliefs. I do not endorse any specific religion in this book, but I do support connecting with something greater than yourself. Connecting with a higher power is something that I learned through the Twelve Steps program—a set of spiritual principles for life and recovery—first published in the *Big Book* of Alcoholics Anonymous.

I choose to call my higher power God, and I use the pronouns *he* and *him*. However, I understand and embrace some people's use of feminine pronouns. When you see *God* and related words in this book, translate them into whatever names or concepts have meaning for you.

Good-Bye Ed, Hello Me is for you regardless of where you are on recovery road or even if you have not set foot on the path yet. If you have ever heard Ed whisper in your ear—even just flirtatious little remarks such as "You need to lose a few pounds"—this book is for you. It is for you regardless of your age, ethnicity, gender, or specific eating disorder diagnosis (or lack thereof). While I obviously speak from a female perspective, my goal in writing this book has been to make it accessible to men as well. This goal was inspired by the many brave men I have met who battle eating disorders and have shared their stories with me.

This book will inspire and guide you, but it will not save you. You are the only one who can do that. One of the most important ways is by getting professional help from people who are trained in treating eating disorders. Both outpatient and inpatient treatment can be expensive, and most people have at least some difficulty affording it. (I sure did.) I have heard people say, "Get professional help if you can afford it, and get professional help if you can't afford it." In other words, do whatever it takes to get it. (See the Resources section in the back of this book for guidance.)

With the help of a therapist, you can build a strong support team that includes not only your therapist but also a dietitian, doctors, and other necessary health care professionals, as well as trusted friends and family members. Always be honest with your support team. I have received e-mails from people who have hidden their eating disorder from their spouses, children, and others for twenty years or more. These people finally experienced healing when they got real help and broke through the secrecy and shame.

I have been happily surprised to learn that treatment professionals assign *Life Without Ed* as reading material to families and friends, who find it helpful to get inside the mind of someone with an eating disorder. This book can help your loved ones in the same way, so you might want to pass it along to your mom, spouse, or someone else after you finish it. Or read it a second time with your therapist or support group.

You might have chosen to pick up this book after reading *Life Without Ed*, but I wrote *Good-Bye Ed, Hello Me* to stand on its own. If you do decide to read both books, you can do so in any order or both at the same time.

As with *Life Without Ed*, I've organized this book in such a way that you can approach it however you choose. The short sections are ideal for digesting a little information from time to time. You can use this book as a reference guide and carry it with you, keep it by your bed and read a little each night, or do something else. There is no right or wrong way.

Also similar to my first book, you will find humor here, because I have found that laughter really is one of the best medicines. I never would have recovered from my eating disorder or other serious (that is, not a laughing matter) issues in my life had I not learned how to laugh—and done it a lot. Laughter helps us put things in perspective, giving us the hope to move forward.

You will find practical exercises scattered throughout this book in sections titled "Real Action." I have learned in my personal growth work that changes really start happening when I actually do something. Thinking about concepts and techniques is helpful, but action is what makes the difference. Grab your journal or just a pen and some paper and give the exercises that resonate with you (the ones that you think will make a difference in your life) an honest effort. Talk about your work with your therapist.

While *Life Without Ed* guides you to a divorce from Ed, *Good-Bye Ed, Hello Me* takes you from the divorce (and helps you make it final) to a connection with yourself—to an inner marriage of mind, body, and spirit. The seven parts of the book are even set up to mirror this inner marriage. We recover from our eating disorders and recover ourselves.

Because I am now divorced from Ed (and married to myself), my entire support system in life has changed. In *Life Without Ed*, I talked a lot about the professionals who made up my treatment team—my psychotherapist, Thom Rutledge, LCSW (who taught me about the metaphor of Ed); my dietitian; and my doctors. In this book, I make references to that team, but I don't actually work with them anymore and haven't for many years. I am very grateful that these folks tirelessly supported me along recovery road and also helped me to move on to my own path in life.

I have moved on from the therapy group that I talked about in *Life Without Ed* as well. Looking back, I can see how truly lucky I was to be part of a group made up of people who really wanted to get better. (We were not always succeeding, but we wanted to be.) If we hadn't, I wouldn't have been a part of the group for so long. I have not attended group therapy for more years than I can remember, and I actually don't connect much with those women anymore. We have gone on with our lives—graduating from school, starting families, and other exciting things. We have drifted apart for the best reason I can think of—we are truly living!

Treatment for my eating disorder was a strange thing, because the goal was ultimately to get better and discontinue treatment, which oftentimes meant ending relationships that had become very important to me. This was scary. I was sometimes afraid to get better, because I did not want to have to quit going to therapy or to group. Luckily, all along the way, I was building the foundation for my new, Ed-free life.

My support in life today includes my family, my friends in Nashville and other parts of the world, and close work colleagues. Therapy was so beneficial to me during recovery that I use it as a source of support for life as well. Since recovering from my eating disorder, I have seen several different therapists, but for simplicity's sake, in this book, I combine them into the persona of "Ann."

People struggling with eating disorders have asked me over and over in my work, "Does it *really* get better?" Yes, it does. Your therapist, dietitian, doctors, friends, family members, and others would not encourage you to work so hard in recovery if it did not ultimately get better—*really* better. I would not encourage you to go through the sweat, blood, and tears of the recovery process only to reach some kind of mediocre state where you were just "managing" the illness. It is possible to live without Ed.

No one wants to go through life walking on eggshells around food, and you don't have to. In fact, you don't have to walk on eggshells in your life. Eating disorders are not really about food and weight anyway, so recovery is not just about food and weight. It is about much more.

If you are anything like me, after overcoming an eating disorder—possibly the toughest battle you will ever face—other things that pop up in your life will not seem nearly as challenging. You will have the strength to climb mountains and reach for the sky.

Recovery is not just about breaking away from Ed; it is also about falling in love with life. Like I said earlier, you can think of it as getting divorced from Ed and getting married to yourself. You won't need a white dress, pink roses, or a three-tiered wedding cake. (There is absolutely nothing wrong with cake though!) You won't have to wear white satin shoes to walk down this path—your own path. All you need for this celebration is you. Celebrate you. Celebrate your life.

Ed sure won't like all of this celebrating, especially when he is not invited to the party. When you are fighting him along the way and it sometimes feels like you are falling apart, remember that you are really coming together.

In the process, you will find yourself. You will build healthy relationships. You will have the strength to get out of bad ones. Like me, you might even skip your first marriage. Just think of it as skipping your first divorce too.

Skip as many marriages as you want. Skip some pages in this book. Skip in the parking lot. Just don't skip out on life. Jump into your life. Run toward your dreams. Reach out and find yourself. Say a big good-bye to Ed and say an even bigger "Hello me!"

I thank God for my handicaps, for through them, I have found myself, my work and my God.

—HELEN KELLER

1

HAPPILY DIVORCED

Life Without Ed

In order to divorce Ed, I needed a recovery toolbox stocked with tools that really worked. Even more important than having the tools, I needed to actually use them. Finding a life without Ed meant consistently applying what I learned in treatment to each step of my recovery journey. It meant facing the food. When I fell down along the way, I had to get back up again. Part 1 will take you back to the basics of eating disorder recovery and reinforce what works and what doesn't. Get ready to take some real action.

Recovered (Period.)

"I'M JENNI. I have an eating disorder," I said as we went around the room introducing ourselves in a Twelve Step meeting. As I spoke the words "I have an eating disorder," I felt a knot in the pit of my stomach. I felt like I was lying to myself and to everyone else. I thought, "I don't have an eating disorder. Why did I just say that?"

I said it to fit in with the standard format of the Twelve Step meeting. John had begun, "I'm John. I have an eating disorder." Then Sue: "I'm Sue. I have an eating disorder."

So I just followed suit, but I won't do it again. That phrase may fit in with the format of the meeting, but it sure does not fit into my life. From now on, I will say, "I am Jenni. I am recovered from an eating disorder."

It took years and years of hard work, energy, and pain to get myself to the place where that statement is true. I did not work for almost a decade to walk around saying that I still have an eating disorder when I don't.

My personal experience is that I must speak my truth, claim what is true for me: I am recovered. I don't still have an eating disorder, and I am not always going to be in recovery. I refuse to give Ed any power in my life today. Looking back, I can see how he used that kind of power to stay in my life for far too long. I can also see that defining myself in terms of my illness was a self-fulfilling prophecy. As long as I believed Ed was waiting around every corner to get me, guess what? He was waiting around every corner to get me.

Sure, there were many points when I was "in recovery," and checking in at a Twelve Step meeting with "I have an eating disorder" suited me just fine. Those were times when I was still acting out with eating disordered behaviors or when I was consumed by the fear of relapse.

I am grateful that people who had been through it themselves told me, "It is possible to be fully recovered from an eating disorder." Knowing that in recovery could become fully recovered was pivotal in my life, so I like to offer that same hope to others today.

Many people out there are at the same place I am in regard to their eating disorder, but they prefer to keep saying that they are in recovery as opposed to being recovered. They believe that the moment they say they are recovered is the moment they will relapse. The phrase *in recovery* reminds them that life is a process and that there is always room to grow. Of course, an important part of my being recovered encompasses this life growth as well, so you might be thinking that this is all a lot of semantics.

To further confuse you, a friend of mine who's in recovery from alcoholism and an eating disorder actually uses both terms. She says that she works a recovery program daily and is thus in recovery. But quoting the *Big Book* of Alcoholics Anonymous, she also says that she is "recovered from a hopeless condition of mind and body."

The point is, semantics or not, we all must figure out for ourselves how we define freedom. If saying what I say—"I am recovered"—feels wrong to you, say something else. I can't force my vision on you and vice versa. When you are alone and grounded, what feels best to you? Do what works.

Claim your truth, and I will claim mine. "I'm Jenni. I'm recovered from an eating disorder."

Real Action: Your Vision of Freedom

When you have some alone time, sit quietly and take a few deep breaths. After you feel grounded, write answers to the following questions:

1. Does using the term *in recovery* keep me sick or keep me healthy?
2. Does using the term *recovered* keep me sick or keep me healthy?
3. Look at your responses to questions 1 and 2. What is your vision of freedom from Ed? Post your vision in a prominent place in your home.

I Am Different

W HEN I WALKED into group therapy for the first time, I
scanned the room to see how different I was from everyone
else. I quickly determined that I was fatter than all of the other
women. I continued to find more and more differences, both real
and perceived. "I am different" was my anthem.

Are you different too? Maybe you are a man in treatment with
mostly women. Maybe you are an older person in treatment with
mostly younger people. Eating disorders do not discriminate by
gender, age, sexual orientation, culture, ethnicity, social class,
financial status, or anything else.

Or have you received the diagnosis of eating disorders not otherwise specified (EDNOS) and feel like you don't have a "real"
eating disorder? Many people with EDNOS have told me they feel
this way. The truth is that EDNOS *is* a real eating disorder that
can be just as dangerous as anorexia and bulimia; it currently
includes the diagnosis of binge eating disorder (BED)—a life-
threatening disorder in itself. We all might do different things
with food, but we all use food in an unhealthy way (that is, until
we recover).

I don't pay a lot of attention to specific diagnostic criteria,
because I know that people can use this information to disqualify
themselves from treatment. I used to think, "I don't binge enough
to have bulimia," or "I haven't lost enough weight to have
anorexia."

I don't even mention certain eating disordered behaviors,
because I don't want to trigger similar behaviors in others. So if
you read this book and think, "Jenni never mentions [insert your
choice of eating disordered behavior here], so I must not have an
eating disorder," think again. I probably didn't mention that par-

ticular behavior for a reason. Most likely, it was a dangerous behavior that I had learned about by reading a book, so I am careful not to talk about it.

You might feel that you are different because you don't know your diagnosis and believe that your eating behaviors might not be severe enough to warrant one. An eating disorder is an illness that tells us we don't have the illness, and that aspect of it (denial) keeps many of us alone. If food and weight make your life unmanageable, if you are just functioning and not truly living, then you deserve help.

Maybe you don't believe you deserve it, because you have not undergone the same level of trauma as other people. I have learned that trauma is relative to the person experiencing it. What might not seem traumatic to someone else could be very real and traumatic to you.

Or is it that you look physically normal and are not underweight or overweight? Eating disorders come in all shapes and sizes, every number on the scale. I was at some of my worst points with Ed when I looked normal.

My point here is that we are all different. I proved early on that I was different, and I tried to use that as an excuse for why I could not get better. I thought that therapy might work for others, but it wouldn't work for me because I was different. I was afraid of possibly failing at something that worked for others. It was easier to be different than to fail.

It was also easy to use being different as an excuse to slip off into isolation: "No one in my therapy group understands me, so why should I even go? My 'normal' friends don't get me, so why should I hang out with them?" I left myself out of humanity by focusing on differences. This isolation only strengthened Ed.

To ultimately recover, I had to begin seeking similarities. I learned to do this by following the lead of people in my therapy group. I remember one woman who didn't complain about feeling fat like the rest of us. Instead she complained specifically about feeling full. Instead of focusing on how she was different from us, she would say, "I might not feel fat, but I do feel full. It's the same intolerable type of feeling. Just like you guys, I will do anything to make it go away." She would also do anything to recover.

I learned by example to identify rather than compare. I consider comparing a cruel form of punishment. (Remember the phrase "compare and despair.") I would say cruel and unusual, but unfortunately, in our society, comparisons are not unusual. They seem to be the norm. If you are like me and insist on being different, be different by not comparing and by seeking similarities.

You are neither worse nor better than anyone else. You are unique—just like everyone else. Choose to think differently.

Back to the Basics

"I'M HOPELESS. I will never recover." I said this throughout early recovery. I said it to anyone who would listen, and I especially said it to everyone on my treatment team (many times over). Oftentimes, one of them would look at me and say, "Who are you?"

By this time, I had been in recovery for months, so I knew they hadn't just forgotten my name. That said, playing along with their little game, I would say, "I'm Jenni." After a while, I knew where the game was going—to their response, "No, that wasn't Jenni talking. That was Ed."

Soon enough, people in my therapy group, friends, and family members all started playing the game too. I didn't think this game was much fun and, in fact, became rather frustrated with it. While I wallowed in self-pity about how hopeless I was with Ed, people seemed to want me to take responsibility for my own recovery. (The nerve of them. I mean, really!)

They wanted me to separate from Ed and understand that he was the one saying, "You are hopeless. You will never recover." Ed is a thief, and he likes to steal the *I* pronoun. He changes "*You* are hopeless" and "*You* will never recover" to "*I* am hopeless. *I* will never recover."

As long as he could get me to change *you* to *I*—and get me to believe that those thoughts were coming from me and not him—then he could win. Ed's existence relies heavily on the fact that you forget to separate from him (and forget everything else you learn in recovery as well). One of his greatest tactics is amnesia.

So one of the basics of recovery for me was to remember to separate. At one point, I even posted notes all over my home that said, "Separate, separate, separate." (I'm not sure what my landlord thought about my home decor.) While I was practicing separating myself from Ed, I still sometimes agreed with and obeyed him. This was actually progress in the beginning, because I at least was remembering to separate. A conversation sometimes went like this:

Agreeing and Obeying

ED: You can't survive without me. You need me.

JENNI: Maybe I should at least try to leave you.

ED: Don't even think about it. Without me, you'd be a big, fat nobody.

JENNI: Okay, you're probably right. I won't try.

As I gained more strength in recovery, I learned to disagree with Ed, but sometimes I still obeyed him. Despite this compliance, I was making progress. Here's the scene:

Disagreeing, Still Obeying

ED: You can't survive without me. You need me.

JENNI: I don't need you, Ed. I have learned that in recovery.

ED: Don't even think about leaving. Without me, you'd be a big, fat nobody.

JENNI: That's not true, but I'm scared to leave you now. So I'll stay.

To recover, I not only had to separate from Ed and disagree with him, I also needed to disobey him. To get this independence from Ed, I had to become more dependent on my support team. I had to trust them and let them love me. (I couldn't love myself yet.) I began to pick up the phone and call for help. When I called someone, I had to make sure that I actually put myself, not Ed, on the line. These days, people find text messaging a helpful way to get support, but Ed knows how to text, so make sure all of the messages are from you and not from him.

My conversations with Ed began to look more like this:

Disagreeing and Disobeying
ED: You can't survive without me. You need me.
JENNI: I don't need you, Ed. I have learned that in recovery.
ED: Don't even think about leaving. Without me, you'd be a big, fat nobody.
JENNI: That's not true, and I will leave you. Just watch me!

What I ultimately discovered is that it was possible for me to disobey Ed even if I agreed with him. For instance, for a long time during recovery, I believed Ed when he told me I was fat, but I still disobeyed him by eating what I was supposed to eat. This was the kind of power move that helped make our divorce final.

It turns out that I wasn't hopeless, and I am recovered. Guess what? You're not hopeless, and you can recover too.

Real Action: Making the Split from Ed

One of the best exercises to help me break away from Ed was creating a back-and-forth dialogue with him in my journal. Practice dialoging with Ed by writing out what Ed says to you and how you respond. The purpose of this exercise is simply to practice separating from Ed—whether you disagree with him or not.

Ed: _____
You: _____
Ed: _____
You: _____

A few important things to remember:

- *Don't let Ed steal the* I.
- *Don't let him have the last word.* In my earlier examples, notice that I always had the last word. Even if I agreed with Ed, I still took some power back by giving myself the final say.
- *Practice. Practice. Practice.* With continued practice separating from Ed, you will gain the strength required to disagree with and disobey him on a regular basis.

Normal Eating?

ORMAL EATING WAS an oxymoron to me—like "clear as mud." *Normal* and *eating* seemed to be contradictory terms. I had manipulated food for so long that my eating was anything but ordinary. Abnormal eating actually seemed normal to me. To fully recover, I had to find a new normal—a balanced approach.

Since our bodies are built differently, my normal might not be yours. I found mine through intuitive eating, which is an approach described in the book *Intuitive Eating* by Evelyn Tribole, M.S., RD, and Elyse Resch, M.S., RD, FADA.

This mindful and moderate approach does not include label reading, calorie counting, or rigid rules. (Obviously, Ed is not a big fan of intuitive eating.) It is about getting in touch with your hunger and fullness cues—eating when you are hungry and stopping when you are full. At the same time, it is flexible, a nondiet approach that includes eating foods that you crave and truly enjoy.

Intuitive eating is about making peace with food. Unlike what Ed teaches us, food does not have a moral value like good or bad. In other words, your worth as a person does not depend on whether or not you eat a so-called bad food. Food should not be labeled good or bad, safe or unsafe, healthy or unhealthy. Food is just food. In the name of eating healthy, people can get so focused on eating only organic or all-natural foods that they become dangerously malnourished. *Orthorexia* is the unofficial term for an eating disorder characterized by this type of unhealthy obsession with "healthy" eating.

I'm sure that I ate intuitively as a baby, but I don't remember that. The earliest age I can recall is four years old, and I did not trust my body even then. So as far back as I can remember, food had some sort of power over me.

Treatment professionals and others often tried to help me understand intuitive eating by saying, "Think back to a time when you had a balanced relationship with food." I felt hopeless, thinking, "There was no such time." I had no memories of this type of eating in my own life, but when I started on the recovery path, I learned how to do it anyway.

I did not begin intuitive eating on day one of recovery. It would have been impossible for me at this point, because I had lost touch with my hunger and fullness cues. I remember complaining a lot about how people wanted me to eat when I didn't feel hungry. At lunchtime, I would say, "I'm not hungry. It still feels like breakfast is sitting in my stomach." I learned that part of this sensation had to do with the fact that restrictive eating had caused the movement of food through my digestive system to slow down, causing a false feeling of fullness. I would say, "I'm still full. I don't need to eat." But the truth was that I did need to eat. Eating was how I was going to become healthy and eventually get in touch with my body signals. (During this process of learning how to eat again, I was under a doctor's care to make sure my body was responding appropriately.)

Because I was initially disconnected from my body, I began my path to intuitive eating with a food plan prescribed by my dietitian. I ate a specific amount of food at certain times every day. This meant filling out a little form listing what I ate and taking it to my weekly dietary appointment. It also meant gradually increasing the amount of food and slowly introducing new foods, so I didn't eat the same combinations of things every day. I had to take time out of my schedule to go grocery shopping, and to support myself through this potentially triggering experience, I sometimes took trusted people with me. After I had made significant progress working with a meal plan, I moved toward intuitive eating.

With help along the way from my support team, I began to trust my body. I fell down more times than I can count, but I got up and kept going. I am finally an intuitive eater. (Learn more about this process in "What if I Never Stop Eating?" in Part 5.) Today I can tell what my body wants to eat and when. It is actually kind of fun. By listening to my body, I can decipher whether I want a brownie, a cookie, or something altogether different, like a turkey sandwich. For the most part, I eat when I'm hungry and stop when I'm full. When I'm at my parents' house, I sometimes eat more than usual because my mom's food just tastes so good. (She actually makes her own piecrust!) Intuitive eating is imperfect and flexible like this. I don't worry when I eat an extra slice of my mom's apple pie, because I trust my body. Unlike what Ed used to tell me, when I have eaten too much, I don't need to compensate by restricting during the next meal. Also, despite what Ed says, one slice of pie won't cause me to gain weight overnight.

I am finally spontaneous with food; I no longer have to be rigid about what or when I eat. When I go out to a restaurant, I order what I really want. Sometimes I eat cake for breakfast, because it happens to be in the house and it sounds good. Foods that once caused me to binge are no longer triggers. Building up to this freedom was a snail-paced process. It didn't happen all in one day or even in one year.

I am finally a normal eater. I can now see how *normal* and *eating* go together. It's all as clear as mud.

The Missing Piece

DON'T LOOK ANY further. It is here at last! The missing piece has been found. This is the section that should have appeared somewhere around page 12 in *Life Without Ed*. Better late than never, it is on this page of this book. This important idea might upset you. It did me, but here goes.

Don't blame Ed for anything. When I first began to make the split from Ed, I made the mistake of blaming him for my destructive behaviors with food. Here's the scene:

> **ED:** Jenni, go to Wendy's tonight and binge.
> **JENNI:** Okay, I'll do it. (And I would.)

Later, I would call someone in my therapy group and say, "I binged last night, but Ed made me do it. I had no choice." Inevitably, this person would tell me that I did have a choice. In one way or another, people told me over and over to stop blaming Ed and to start being accountable for my own recovery. Needless to say, these moments were not those warm and fuzzy ones that I liked having so much with the people in my therapy group; they were hard truths to face.

As soon as I recognized that Ed existed separate from me, my job was to respond to what he said. If he said to binge, I had to decide whether or not I was going to binge. Maybe I couldn't control what he said or did, but I could sure take responsibility for my own actions. Ed didn't have to change—I did.

Apparently—and I understand this now—the point of personifying Ed is to take personal responsibility, not to blame. The point of my working so hard to separate from Ed was so that I could make room for my own opinion and become the decision maker in my own life, to separate his voice from my own and give myself the power to choose between the two. The metaphor was a tool that gave me the power to choose recovery. The choice was all mine, not Ed's.

This information may still be missing from *Life Without Ed*, but you are responsible for making sure that it is no longer missing from your life. You can blame me for forgetting to mention this concept until now. But you can't blame Ed for anything—not anymore.

Kath

I T WAS A Sunday morning in March. My phone rang. I recognized the number on the caller ID and was afraid it was the call I had hoped never to receive. I answered anyway. And I was right.

On the other end of the phone, Kath's mom said, "We lost her."

My dear friend Kath had died from the devastating effects of an eating disorder at forty-one years old. I had met Kath a few years earlier when I helped her find treatment for an eating disorder she had battled since her early twenties. She had been in and out of treatment centers for years, but this time, she wanted to get better more than ever.

In that moment on the phone with Kath's mom, all of the facts about eating disorders that I had known intellectually to be true became real: Eating disorders are real, life-threatening illnesses. Anorexia has the highest mortality rate of any psychiatric disorder. These facts were now more than just words on some website. They represented my friend and the deep pain left behind in the hearts of her family and friends.

Tears streaming down my face, I thought about my last conversation with Kath. I had told her that I was afraid her mom was going to call me one day and say the very words that she essentially did. I asked Kath specifically what I could do to help, saying that my previous attempts obviously were not working. I asked how her appointments with her doctors were going. I told her that I loved her and to call me anytime. Her mom called that Sunday, but Kath never did.

Why didn't she call? Why does someone so young have to die? Why hadn't we all done more? What could we have done differently? I now know these are questions often asked by people in the same situation.

That same day, I received a call from a woman named Melissa who was struggling with an eating disorder. She said, "I want to die. I don't want to live anymore." After just losing my friend, I had no patience for someone who wanted to die. I thought about Kath and said, "Melissa, right now, I want to talk to the part of you that wants to live." After all, that was the part that had decided to pick up the phone and call me. Even if it was undetectable to Melissa at the time, I wanted to talk to that part. We had to find her motivation to recover.

One of the many things I learned from Kath is that there is a part inside each of us that wants to live. Even though Kath's eating disorder controlled most of her behaviors around food, even though she was never able to let it go, there was always a part of her that desperately wanted to live, that wanted freedom. Even though this part might have been small at times, it always gave her hope.

When you feel like you would rather die than live another day with an eating disorder, know that I used to feel that way too. Search deep inside yourself for the part that wants to live. It's the part that made you open this book and start reading. It's the part that pushes you to go to therapy.

Your motivation to recover might be small in the beginning. Right now, maybe you are not even in recovery for yourself, but for your spouse or kids. Or maybe your reason for getting help is so that you can attend college next semester. People might tell you "If you don't do it for yourself, you won't get better." I disagree. So does my good friend and colleague, Michael E. Berrett, Ph.D., coauthor of *Spiritual Approaches in the Treatment of Women with Eating Disorders*. He says, "Embrace not just any reason to recover, but every reason. Over time, you will eventually understand and embrace one of the best reasons to recover—that you are worth it."

Ed will use every possible reason he can to hold you by his side. (If your dog runs away, Ed will tell you to binge. If someone you know is diagnosed with a serious illness, Ed will tell you to restrict.) So you must use every reason you can to break free of him as well.

Do whatever it takes to get the professional help you need. An eating disorder is a global attack on your body, negatively affecting every part, from the hair on your head to the tip of your toes. No organ is spared. The reality is that without treatment, this illness is terminal. I look back at my life with Ed and see clearly how I could have died. At the time, I thought I was young and invincible. Today I see that I was just lucky. In some ways, an eating disorder is like Russian roulette. It is gambling with your life. You never know when your body is just going to give out without warning. And if the disorder does not take your body, it will kill your spirit. Don't let it.

Kath lost her battle, but we are all still in the game. That Sunday in March, Melissa found the part of her that wanted to live.

Kath's dream was to share her story and help others struggling with eating disorders. Her story lives on. Thank you, Kath.

Real Action: Motivate Yourself

We often write in our journals when we are feeling bad and not doing too well. I encourage you to make an extra effort to write in your journal when you are feeling good. When you experience a good day in recovery (or even just a good hour), write about it. Describe how you feel, how you arrived at that place. Begin to write more and more journal entries that talk about how recovery is a real possibility for you. You might want to tag these entries in your journal or even start a separate journal for this.

Then when you are not feeling particularly motivated, read these journal entries and discover how recovery is a reality for you. Your journal comes from you, so it is the most powerful book you have. You know yourself better than I or any other author can.

*Journal

Ana, Mia, Ed, and Helga

IT ALWAYS WORKED for my eating disorder to be a man named Ed. Treating it like an abusive husband who was controlling and manipulative worked for me. Ed sometimes acted like the "sweet" husband who tried to keep me under his control by showering me with gifts. But sometimes he was the loud, screaming abuser who would forcibly knock me to the ground. People from across the globe have connected with the metaphor of Ed.

And that is all this is—a metaphor. Of course, my eating disorder was never really a guy named Ed who followed me around night and day, but it sure felt like it. Ed stood for a collection of beliefs I had learned since I was born. Unlike other recovery models, I learned that Ed was not an aspect of my authentic self, so my goal was always to separate from him. Different recovery models and tools work better for different people.

It doesn't matter what you call your eating disorder, whether male or female, as long as it works for you. Call your eating disorder Tom, Nancy, or Linda if those names fit best. My friend, Carrie Arnold, coauthor of *Next to Nothing*, called her eating disorder Helga at one time. A guy I know calls his eating disorder Mia— short for *bulimia*.

I just received a MySpace message from a young woman named Mary Lynn, who talks about Ana, obviously for *anorexia*. You might find, like Mary Lynn, that your eating disorder changes its identity depending on the specific situation. She wrote, "He is literally disguising himself. When I am trying hard to fight for recovery, he is Ed. However, when I am in a weak moment and want to hang on to my eating disorder, he changes to Ana. While Ed is not my friend, Ana still is. She promises to make me happy and thin.

"As Ana, I have realized that Ed is just disguising himself as a more appealing figure, an old friend who is 'only there to help.' But Ana and Ed are one and the same! There is really no Ana at all. It is just Ed trying to get in my bedroom door. What a stinker he is! He had me fooled. But you know what? I'm not letting him in. Not anymore!"

Mary Lynn's eating disorder is female (Ana) when it tries to appear friendly and male (Ed) when it is overtly controlling and abusive. The important point is that she recognizes the differences and is standing up for herself, taking responsibility for her recovery regardless of the specific names.

If speaking in metaphorical language like this doesn't work for you, by all means, just call your illness "eating disorder." Work with your therapist to find or even create a model of recovery that fits well with your life. Using metaphors is just a means to the end we are all seeking: freedom.

Your Science Lesson

A BOOK ABOUT EATING disorders is not complete without talking about science. I have a Bachelor of Science degree in biochemistry, but I am not a biochemist. So get ready for your amateur science lesson. Class is about to begin!

I have heard debate after debate in the eating disorder field about genes versus jeans. Are eating disorders caused by biological (genes) or cultural (jeans) factors? One of my former doctors and renowned expert in the field, Ovidio Bermudez, M.D., says "It's not genes *or* jeans; it's genes *and* jeans." Leading researcher Cynthia Bulik, Ph.D., agrees: "Genes load the gun, but environment pulls the trigger." Researchers don't believe there is a specific eating disorder gene, but rather that people inherit a latent vulnerability that can lead to the development of such a disorder.

Dr. Bulik's quote is an accurate fit to my personal experience. I believe that I inherited the genetic vulnerability for an eating disorder in the form of personality traits like anxiety, compulsivity, and perfectionism. This was genetics loading the gun. I think the main part of the environment that pulled the trigger for me was living in a Western culture that puts too much focus on the ideal of thinness. (When I restricted food to achieve the thin ideal, dieting became an eating disorder.) Other environmental aspects can include life experiences, peer relationships, family issues, and more.

A well-known study conducted in the Fiji Islands by Anne E. Becker, M.D., Ph.D., Sc.M., clearly shows how genes and environment interact in regard to culture. Prior to 1995, there was no talk of dieting or calories in Fiji. In fact, women wanted to be robust in both body and appetite. In 1995, American television was introduced with, of course, images of very thin American women. After just three years of television watching, dieting had become popular, with 11 percent of Fijian girls vomiting to control their weight. The gene pool did not change, but the environment did. One explanation is that those individuals with a greater genetic vulnerability for an eating disorder found that their attempts at dieting quickly became the first steps on the path to illness.

I think it is important to note that the Fijian girls were not really trying to be thin for the sake of being thin. They wanted to be thin to be like the American women on television who appeared successful, with great jobs and lots of money. Taking this into account, I can see that it wasn't necessarily the idea of thinness that I wanted either. What I wanted was what I believed came with thinness. The media had taught me that to be thin was to be popular, smart, happy, and successful. That's what I wanted. If the media had told me that people with purple hair were the popular, smart, happy, and successful ones, guess who would have had the brightest purple shade of hair possible?

At the end of the day, how does science help us? Well-known expert Craig Johnson, Ph.D., believes that science is crucial in prevention. We know eating disorders run in families, and we also know they often develop around puberty. To families who have been touched by an eating disorder (meaning someone in the family has already been diagnosed), Dr. Johnson says, "Be on the lookout when other children in the family enter puberty. They should be discouraged from dieting and high-risk activities." (A high-risk activity is one that encourages weight loss and/or excessive exercise, including modeling, ballet, gymnastics, and cross-country running.) Dieting and a high-risk activity combined with a genetic vulnerability could send an individual into a full-fledged eating disorder.

For a while, this idea of eating disorders running in families terrified me. I even told people that I would never have kids, because I wouldn't want to bring a child into the world who would suffer with an eating disorder. Now I can see things more clearly. Maybe my child would be at greater risk for an eating disorder, but I also have great tools for prevention. Because I know the risks involved, as Dr. Johnson mentions, I could actually help keep my child from ever developing the illness in the first place. (Needless to say, if I ever have a daughter, she might not twirl around in ballet slippers, but she might hit a softball out of the park.)

All in all, science has taught me that eating disorders really are life-threatening illnesses, not simply lifestyle choices. Neither sufferers nor families are to blame. Eating disorders are complex biopsychosocial illnesses that cannot be traced specifically to any one cause.

Does the "bio" component of eating disorders mean that I will never be fully recovered? Will I be eating disordered forever? If you are at this point in the book, I'm sure you know my answer to that. Absolutely not!

I was not born with an eating disorder. I was born with a genetic vulnerability. Western society taught me to apply certain personality traits in a negative way—a way that led to an eating disorder. I learned in recovery to bring these traits to the light instead of the darkness. In other words, I learned to use them in a positive way, which is a concept about which Carolyn Costin is eloquent. She says that anxiety becomes high energy when taken to the light. For me, it worked like this: I used to live in a constant state of anxiety, worrying about the past and the future. Now I do my best to focus my attention on the present moment. So the mental energy I used to waste on worrying is channeled into the present, making me better able to focus intently and enthusiastically on a task (whether work or play). In a similar way, perfectionism becomes tenacity, and compulsivity becomes drive. Traits that once brought us down can lift us up when taken to the light.

I thought it was important to bring all of this science to the light. That's your science lesson for the day. Class dismissed.

✩ My Heart ✩

D O YOU LIKE music by Kelly Clarkson, Rascal Flatts, or the
Beatles? If so, you may own one of their CDs that includes
a hidden track, that song that plays unexpectedly at the end of the
album, sometimes after minutes of silence. I just listened to a CD
that I've had for years and heard the hidden track for the very first
time.

This reminded me of my own internal hidden track, a voice in
my life that was always there but that I didn't pay attention to for
a long time. It took about thirty years of walking (and crawling)
around on the earth for me finally to be still enough mentally and
physically to not only hear but to actually listen to my hidden
track. That track is my intuition.

In therapy, Ann and I have both noticed that when I say something that comes from my intuition, I tend to raise my hand to my
heart. For this reason, I sometimes call my intuition my heart.

Intuition tells us something without facts and figures. It is the
wise voice that says what to do and which way to turn. It is an
inner knowing, a gut feeling or hunch. I believe that my intuition
connects me with God.

When I was struggling with my eating disorder, I rejected my
intuition and listened to Ed's logic. (Now there's an oxymoron—
Ed's logic.) To fully recover, I had to kick him out of the driver's
seat and become my own decision maker.

It took a long time, but I can finally say that Jenni is the decision maker in my life. I call the shots. And I call the best shots
when I connect with my heart. If I go inside, I can usually tell
what my heart is saying these days. When I can't, I often just have
to wait. It wasn't always this easy. It took lots of time and practice

with living in the moment for me to connect more easily with my heart. It took even longer to trust it.

Even today I sometimes don't turn to my heart. I don't listen to my intuition because I don't want to know what I know. I did this with Mark. On our first date, his drinking bothered me, but I didn't face this fact until almost two years later. Not a good call on my part. I put blinders on because I wanted the relationship to work so badly. Ultimately, I listened to my heart and called off the wedding.

I have found that my life goes a lot smoother when I connect with my heart. Just like that hidden track on my CD, my heart has been there all along. I just had to sit still long enough to listen.

And, boy, do I love the song that's playing!

Just Eat (Seriously)

"JUST EAT," WELL-MEANING people say to us during our recovery journey. Coming from someone who has never had an eating disorder and who *can* just eat, these two words do not feel supportive—they can even feel somewhat condescending.

That said, I am here to tell you that ultimately—to be recovered—you *do* have to just eat. I learned this years ago from people who were recovered and would say, "Jenni, just eat your food." They said I had been in recovery long enough and I knew too much not to be eating. Somehow, coming from people who had been there, "just eat" didn't feel rude or unsupportive. It felt like the truth I had been avoiding.

I had tried to steer clear of the eating part of recovery for a long time. I thought that if I just talked enough about food in therapy and group, the urges to binge, purge, and restrict would simply go away. I planned to eat in a balanced way when the urges disappeared and eating became easy. The problem with this plan is that eating becomes easy by eating, not by just talking. I could not have recovered without therapy, support groups, and everything else, but I also could not have gotten better without adding food to the mix.

I have heard doctor after doctor say that food is the best medicine to treat an eating disorder. I didn't take my medicine for years. I thought that I could recover with a halfhearted effort in the food department, as long as I was fully devoted to other aspects of recovery. I was wrong. I was stuck, and I wanted more. To get more, I needed to let go of all my attempts to control food.

There was no way to make this difficult and painful process easy. I won't lie to you and say that it is surprisingly simple if you just write about it in your journal or read the right meditation at mealtimes. Yes, journals and meditations are helpful, but they will not take away the pain. Just as in other parts of recovery, you must walk through it. Before I tackled the food head-on, I looked to other people in recovery who were steps ahead of me for inspiration. I once received the following e-mail from Kayce, a member of my therapy group:

> *I am still struggling with not liking anything I eat. Everything tastes horrible, but I am eating anyway. I'm doing what I am supposed to be doing with food, and it's making me so tired. I hope I don't have to spend the rest of my life following my meal plan and being miserable about it.*

This message might not sound particularly uplifting, but it was to me. Kayce was doing what I knew I needed to be doing. She was eating her food. If she could do it, maybe I could too. Kayce is now recovered with a full, happy life. She got there by continuing to do what she was doing: working hard in therapy *and* eating her food. She just ate. It was as simple and as complicated as that.

This was one of the most frustrating parts of recovery for me: I knew what I needed to do, but I couldn't get myself to do it. Time after time, I chose Ed's quick fix over recovery. Eating consistently in a healthy way seemed impossible, but it wasn't.

When it came to decisions about food, I learned to do what I intellectually knew (from appointments with my dietitian) I needed to do instead of reacting to what I was thinking and feeling in the moment with Ed screaming in my ear. Along the way, I cried, yelled, and stayed closely connected with my support team.

For about one year, I made a commitment to call a woman in my therapy group every day at noon. She didn't even have to answer the phone. I was committed to talking with her or her voice mail each day to report how I was doing with food. Sometimes I had difficulty picking up the phone and asking for support, so having a standing appointment like this ensured that I actually did it. This kind of accountability didn't make the act of eating less painful, but it helped me to actually follow through—to eat the food and feel the feelings.

The more I ate in a healthy way, the easier it became. I think a large part of this had to do with my brain getting proper nourishment. When I was not eating well, my doctor would tell me that I was malnourished and that my thinking wasn't right. I believed *his* thinking wasn't right. After all, I had maintained As in school with an active eating disorder. How could my brain not be functioning properly? Well, now that I am fully recovered, I can see plainly that I had not been thinking clearly when I was sick. (I can also see that school would have been much easier for me had I been eating properly.) For those of you saying, "I'm not thin enough to be malnourished," you can be malnourished at a normal or above-average weight.

I can finally say that food is not a problem for me. I no longer have a love/hate relationship with it, but a balanced one. This became a reality for me when I made the choice to just eat.

When I say, "Just eat," remember that I have been there. I know that *just* equals hard work, time, tears, and determination. If you want to recover fully, feel the pain, feel the fear, and just eat. *Just do it.*

Real Action: Plants and Animals

At the beginning of my recovery, I owned one small plant that only needed water every couple of weeks. Later, I had a Japanese flying fish for a while. Today, looking around my home, I am surrounded by a lot of beautiful plants.

Taking care of other living things helped me take care of myself. As I fed them, I was reminded that I too must be fed on a regular basis. Would I starve my plants or not feed my fish for days on end? No, I wouldn't. I needed to take care of myself as well.

If you are in a position to do so, if you are healthy enough and live in an appropriate environment, consider getting a plant or pet. Start with living things that are small and easy to take care of. (Don't go out and buy a horse or anything like that!) If you already own plants or animals, pay more attention to how you meet their daily needs. Experience joy in seeing another living creature grow and thrive. Use this experience to grow and thrive as an individual.

2

BEING SINGLE

Making It on Your Own

I used to think that I could not possibly live without Ed. I didn't know how to deal with normal emotions or the routine of everyday life without bingeing, purging, and restricting. Sometimes I felt so bad without Ed that I wondered why I had ever broken up with him in the first place. Inevitably, I would let him creep back into my life in some way, shape, or form. To move from in recovery to fully recovered, I had to make a different kind of decision to get better, and I'm finally making it on my own. Part 2 will show you how to do the same.

Who Am I Without Ed?

*W*HO AM I *without Ed? We have been together for so long that I am afraid of what my life might look like without him. What if my life is actually worse without him? Sure, things are not exactly great with him. Okay, I admit that things are horribly miserable with Ed, but at least I'm thin. I would definitely rather be thin and miserable than fat and miserable. What if being recovered just means that I'm going to gain weight and be fat and miserable?*

I used to have all these thoughts. I know that many of you have too, because you have e-mailed them to me and sent me handwritten letters (yes, some people still do that). Still others have asked me these questions at presentations. At one time or another, most of us wonder if we can really make it on our own without Ed. We wonder if all this recovery mumbo jumbo is really just that—mumbo jumbo, meaningless talk. We wonder if all the pain and hard work are really worth it in the end. We wonder and we wonder, and then we wonder some more.

What I have discovered is that we can wonder all we want as long as we are still taking steps along recovery road. We can walk and wonder at the same time. In fact, I wondered all these things all the way to that place I call recovered. For me, recovery was a big leap of faith. I held on to lots of hope. I hoped that recovered actually existed. I hoped it was a great place, but I wasn't so sure. I wondered and wondered, but I still kept walking, still had faith that life could be better. I wasn't sure until I got here. But now I'm here, fully recovered. Now I know the answers to those questions.

Yes, recovery is worth all the hard work. No, I am not just fat and miserable. In fact, I am happier than ever before, and I love my body. No, I am not as thin as I used to be, but I don't want to be. My life without Ed is so much better than my life with him that I don't even know how to express it. In my original draft, I wrote that my life is a million times better, but it is actually much better than that.

I finally know who I am without Ed, and I learn more and more about myself every day. I will never stop learning. Some of the things I have learned: I am funnier than I thought; I am more intuitive than I believed. I am more in love with life than I ever imagined possible. The list goes on and on.

If you are still in that wondering ("Who am I without Ed?") phase, you might not be able to fully grasp what I'm saying here. I know I couldn't when I was in your shoes. Like me, you will have to take that leap of faith that recovery is going to be worth it for you. Even though I've been through it, I know I cannot completely convince you right now—no one was able to convince me. But you will get there and experience it for yourself if you keep walking. Then you will know. So keep on walking and wondering. Walk and wonder all the way to freedom.

God Hates Me?

G OD SITS UP in the clouds keeping track of how many mistakes I make on a scorecard—at least I used to think so. If I made too many mistakes, well, I knew where I was headed.

Growing up, I went to church with my family every Sunday, and one of the beliefs I took away was that God was vengeful, wrathful, and punishing. I don't think the rest of the people in my family or even in the church necessarily held this belief, but I sure did. I listened carefully to what I heard during church and took everything literally. I never shared my thoughts with others, never gave myself the opportunity to ask questions or develop another opinion. Needless to say, I was a good little girl who felt guilty a lot of the time.

Even though I feared God and his disapproval, I also believed that he was loving and forgiving (I heard this in church too). I did feel close to him. I prayed every night and meant it. I believed God was listening to what little ol' me had to say.

Gradually Ed crept into my life, pushing God out of the way. When being thin was my focus, there wasn't as much room for God, and he became less and less important, almost as if thinness itself became my object of worship. In a sense, my eating disorder was my higher power. I still prayed like I was supposed to, but I didn't feel anything. As I grew further and further away from God, he seemed less loving and more critical.

I began to feel judged and unworthy. I thought, "Why me? Why do bad things happen to me? Why do I have an eating disorder?" The eating disorder became my evidence that I was not good enough for a higher power to love. The loving, forgiving aspects of God went out the window, as Ed encouraged me to focus on a vengeful, wrathful, and punishing side.

By the time I entered recovery for my eating disorder, I had no connection with God. I didn't even pray anymore. I had a one-sided, unspoken agreement that I would not talk to him. I didn't hate him, but I didn't like him either.

When things with my eating disorder became even worse after I was in recovery, I did hate God. (Or at least, I thought I did.) I thought he hated me too. I was finally fighting Ed, but nothing was getting better. (Ed was mad that I was fighting him, so he became even stronger.) I felt worse than ever, and I blamed God.

In therapy, I was encouraged to keep a "God hates me" journal. I wrote down both my feelings about God and what I thought he felt about me. Through my journal, I began to see inconsistencies in my thinking. For instance, I believed that God loved everyone else in the world, including murderers, but he did not love me. I began to see that this didn't quite make sense. I began to wonder why I was so especially awful. Why was I the one person in the world God hated? Did I really think I was that unique?

I talked with friends who had a level of spirituality I admired. Most of them were in Alcoholics Anonymous. I told them that the God I used to love and talk to now seemed far away. They simply asked, "Who moved?"

I did. God never left. I had not turned to him during challenging times, because I thought that asking him for help was pointless. So I looked to other sources of comfort, wisdom, and understanding—namely, Ed.

I now know that I would have received comfort if I had turned to God instead of to Ed. I would have felt less alone. I would have gained a sense of understanding, a sense of strength. These are all things that Ed had promised to give but failed to deliver. In the end, I got from God what I had wanted from Ed.

I began to pray again. In the beginning, I didn't mean it. As they often say in Twelve Step groups, "I faked it till I made it," and my words eventually began to feel real. I often just said, "God, I am here." I didn't know what else to say, but I was trying. (Trying to pray *is* praying.) Eventually, I started repeating the Serenity Prayer in my head throughout the day:

> *God grant me the serenity to accept the things I cannot change; courage to change the things I can; and wisdom to know the difference.*
>
> —REINHOLD NIEBUHR

Then I began to write my thoughts in a prayer journal in the morning when I woke up or at night before going to bed. Just like when I was a child, I felt as if someone was listening.

I now know that a complete, full life for me means not only saying good-bye to Ed but also saying hello to God. I don't think I would ever have been able to fully love myself without letting God into my life. First I let others love me, then God, and finally I was able to love myself.

I don't know if developing a healthy relationship with a higher power is required to recover from disordered eating, but I do know that it helped me make the leap from always being in recovery to being recovered. I also believe that recovery might have gone more smoothly for me had I found my connection sooner rather than later. I am just grateful that I finally found it.

For a long time, I depended only on my strength in my life. Now I recognize that there is something bigger I can draw on for strength. Today I am more content in the moment and less anxious about tomorrow. I don't fear hell anymore. I've been there.

God opened the gates of hell and invited me to get out. I believe he wants me out of hell and experiencing joy. It turns out that he doesn't hate me after all. He loves me. He loves you too.

Real Action: What Do You Believe?

Sometimes negative experiences make it difficult for us to believe in God or a higher power, which is understandable. On the other hand, we will all end up putting our faith in something or someone. (Many of us have put our faith in Ed.) So why not consider putting our faith in a higher power?

On one side of a sheet of paper, answer this question: "What do you feel when you think about God or a power greater than yourself?" On the other side of the paper, answer this important question: "What do you *want* to feel when you think about God or this higher power?"

Consider discussing your answers with your priest, minister, rabbi, other spiritual leader in your life, or just someone whose spirituality you admire.

Getting to Know Ed

I HAVE OFTEN HEARD that the best way for an alcoholic to find out why he drinks is for him to stop drinking. I discovered why I had an eating disorder when I stopped my destructive behaviors with food. Strangely, we get to know Ed even better when we let him go. We finally gain perspective on him when he's no longer in our face twenty-four hours a day, and we learn what role he has played in our lives and why we've held on to him for so long. If Ed has been acting as a mask for depression, we might feel very low when we first stop bingeing, purging, and starving. I know this from firsthand experience.

Ed definitely had a job in my life. A major role was that he made me feel unique. (For example, Ed would pat me on the back and congratulate me for being the thinnest person in a room.) He also provided comfort by relieving stress and anxiety. These things felt good, and I had to admit and accept that. To say good-bye to Ed, I had to let go of the good as well as the bad. I grieved the good, and that felt bad.

For a long time, I held on to the positive aspects of Ed with a death grip while I tried my best to get rid of the things I hated. Of course, I didn't like how Ed brought exhaustion, physical discomfort, and isolation into my life. I spun my wheels for a long time trying to essentially split Ed in half—get rid of the bad and keep the good. I hit a wall.

To set myself free, I had to say good-bye to all of Ed, the good sides and the bad sides. Getting rid of the bad became more important to me than keeping the good. This meant that I had to stop negotiating with him. When he said, "Sure, Jenni, gain some weight, but only this much," I had to say, "Ed, I will gain as much weight as I need to gain in order to be healthy." The idea of Ed setting my ideal body weight is kind of funny to me now, but that is exactly what I let him do for a long time. It turns out that my ideal body weight is more than Ed hoped for. My ideal body is also healthier and stronger than ever, which is more than I had hoped for. And that's good news!

There is even more good news about losing the good sides of Ed. I learned healthy life coping skills and found my own unique identity. It took me a while, but I found other ways to reduce stress and comfort myself. I no longer needed the benefits Ed had given me because I could get them in my own way, a better way.

So I said good-bye to Ed—the good and the bad—for good.

Jump

I SOMETIMES COMPARE THE recovery process to climbing a tall mountain. Making it to the summit is so difficult that sometimes it seems like a two-steps-forward, three-steps-back kind of process. In other words, recovery is not a straight line; there are setbacks along the way. It takes time and patience to reach the top.

Here comes the tricky part. We assume we are done when we make it to the top. We have worked hard to get there, and we expect to be recovered at that point. But we're not done yet. At the top of the mountain, people hand us a parachute, point to the edge of the cliff, and say, "Jump."

For me, this was when my treatment team said I needed to eat *all* of my food and trust that my body would reach its natural weight. When they said, "Have faith, let go, and trust," I thought they were nuts. I didn't trust them or my body, so I continued to restrict—just a little. I was not bingeing and purging, so I thought I was doing well. A little restricting won't hurt. (This is a common trap!) What I discovered is that a little restricting hurts a lot. It sent me right back down to the foot of the mountain every time. It sent me into relapse.

Lots of other things threw me down the mountain too. I wouldn't jump, so I kept sliding back down to the bottom. I kept relapsing.

I would eventually get sick of the eating disorder and start climbing the recovery mountain all over again. Sometimes it seemed like each climb was getting more and more challenging. I was tired of having to conquer the same barriers over again. I was exhausted and beginning to feel hopeless. Maybe I was the only person who couldn't recover from an eating disorder.

Obviously I wasn't. But what I had to do to fully recover is what all the recovered folks before me did. I had to put the parachute on and jump.

I finally grabbed the parachute and took that leap of faith into the unknown. You might be wondering exactly how I did it. This is one of those parts of recovery that doesn't have a simple explanation. I had to do what my treatment team had been saying: have faith, let go, and trust. This translated into feeling the fear and the pain. I got support from others along the way. I asked people to jump with me, and they said yes.

At first, the free fall was terrifying. Among other things, I wondered, "How much weight will I gain?" and "Will I ever love my new body?" This part was scarier than climbing the mountain. I finally felt the fear, and I gained confidence in the process. I thought, "Maybe I really can do this," and with time, the free fall became exciting. I was free. The struggle with Ed was over. I wouldn't have to climb back up that mountain ever again. What a relief!

I can't emphasize how important it is to put on your metaphorical parachute and jump. Maybe you have done a lot of great work in recovery climbing the mountain, but you haven't jumped yet. So you find yourself relapsing continually, going in and out of treatment centers, or just not getting completely better. You might be an expert on recovery and knowing what you should be doing, but you're not doing it.

Are you stuck in this cycle of trying to avoid the hard part?

If you really do everything that your treatment team tells you, what will happen? Will you really be happy? This is the jumping part.

Jumping is scary, so don't wait around until you're not scared to do it. Jump now and declare independence from Ed. When you don't think you can do it, know that I once felt the same way. And look at me now. I'm still flying!

My New Reality

I WAS A CLOSET drinker. No, I didn't drink closets. I drank diet soda and lots of it. I drank so much diet soda that I was embarrassed for people to know, so I hid it. I hid the empty cans; I hid the full cans. I hid myself when I was buying the cans. I put a lot of energy into hiding my problem and about the same amount of energy into rationalizing that it wasn't really a problem.

Drinking diet soda was a big part of my eating disorder. It gave me a false sense of fullness, and I liked that. Ironically, this behavior that I started in an effort to control the amount of food I ate ultimately contributed to bingeing and other out-of-control behaviors with food.

I was afraid to tell my treatment team about how much of my illness revolved around diet soda. I told them everything else but not this. I held on to this secret weapon with a death grip, and as long as I did, Ed used it as a weapon against me. He used it to keep me trapped in my eating disorder and to disrupt my life. If I went to a vending machine in search of a diet soda and saw a Sold Out sign, I went into panic mode. Could I call myself recovered while simultaneously panicking at a vending machine?

I finally talked with my treatment team and slowly stopped drinking diet sodas. Without the soda to mask my hunger, I ate more, which is what I needed to be doing anyway. I could think more clearly, and I felt healthier. Yes, that particular version of healthy means that I gained some weight too. It meant I was letting go of Ed completely and that my body was finding its natural size.

So I went for a long time without ever touching diet drinks. I wouldn't let myself have even one. Notice the all-or-none thinking. I even had irrational beliefs surrounding diet soda. I thought,

"If someone even sees me near a diet soda, they will think that I am not doing well with my eating disorder." I was terrified of even being near the stuff!

Then, just the other day, I found myself craving a Diet Dr. Pepper, so I walked to the store and bought one. It tasted good, but I felt incredibly guilty.

I confessed to Ann. I told her that I had "slipped" and drank a diet soda. I felt like an alcoholic confessing a relapse. Hanging my head, I said, "I walked to the store and bought a Diet Dr. Pepper yesterday."

Expecting something bigger, she said, "And?"

There was no *and*. I hadn't stolen the soda. I hadn't bought a twelve-pack and drunk it all at once. I hadn't skipped dinner because of the drink. I'd just had a soda. That's all.

"And I actually enjoyed it," I said.

She said, "Maybe your new reality is that you can drink a Diet Dr. Pepper every once in a while."

I jumped in, "But I used to abuse them. I used to . . ."

She cut me off. "I don't want to hear about what used to be. That is your old reality. What is your new reality? Maybe things have changed enough in your life that you can drink an occasional diet soda and just enjoy it."

An interesting idea: my new reality. Ann said that my new reality is that I do not have an eating disorder. I needed to base my decisions on my new reality and not on what used to be. Of course, she talked about accountability as well. She suggested that I just check in with her about the role diet soda is playing in my life. For me, I know that if diet soda actually starts having a role, there could be a problem. If it's just something I drink now and then, there's nothing wrong with that. So far, so good.

This experience with Ann reminded me of how my dietitian had helped me to overcome my fear of binge foods—the specific food items (A, B, and C) that I used to not keep in my house for fear of overeating. If I kept A, B, or C in the house, I would eat all of A, B, or C in one sitting. I had no control, so I avoided them completely. In my new reality, I can keep these foods in my home with no problem at all. I enjoy them in a balanced way.

All in all, I am promoting freedom—not diet soda consumption. I don't want avoiding diet soda to control me as much as drinking it did. I want choices based on my new reality, which includes a balanced mind-set.

Speaking of diet soda, I'm getting kind of thirsty. I think I'll go for water.

Real Action: What Are You Holding On To?

Are you holding on to any eating disordered behaviors? Be honest with yourself about possibly abusive behaviors like gum chewing or drinking too much diet soda, coffee, water, or alcohol. Take a moment to write the truth based on your current reality. Talk with your treatment team about your observations. We are only as sick as our secrets.

I'm Not Wonder Woman

WHEN I WAS a little kid, I was Wonder Woman. Well, I wore Wonder Woman Underoos, and in those moments, I had supernatural powers. When I became too old to wear Underoos, Ed took over the job of giving me supernatural powers. He didn't say that I could leap tall buildings in a single bound or anything like that. No, his powers included not needing food, sleep, people, or fun. They also included being able to work all the time. And you know the rest of that comic strip.

I ended up in treatment. Throughout the recovery process, I tried to keep Ed's supernatural powers, at least some of them. I eventually came to understand that I wouldn't be able to hold on to the not-needing-food part, but I did think that I could hang on to all the rest. I had stopped restricting food, but I was still restricting sleep, people, and fun. I wasn't bingeing on food, but I was bingeing on work.

Despite my best efforts to remain a sleepless, isolated, not-much-fun workaholic living a "recovered" life, I couldn't do it. And trust me when I say that I tried in the most sleepless, isolated, not-much-fun, workaholic kind of way. All of my trying ended with the same result: burnout. I wasn't even thirty, and I was physically and emotionally exhausted most of the time. I was emptying my cup (overworking and not getting enough rest), but I was never filling it up (connecting with people and having fun). I wasn't acting out with eating disordered behaviors, but I was miserable just the same. I wondered, "Is this really recovered?"

No, it wasn't. I had found balance with food, and now I had to find it with life. I couldn't live like I had before, only without Ed. Sooner or later, this type of imbalance in my life would have led me back to him, so I had to change.

Sleep became a requirement. Looking back over my life with Ed, I can see how he used sleep deprivation to keep me under his control. Not sleeping well went hand in hand with not eating well, so sleep had to become a priority in my life. Whether I thought I needed it or not, I had to get enough sleep.

I had to connect with people, genuinely let them into my life. Much of Part 4 of this book talks about how I did that. I also learned how to have fun (see "Having Fun to Save My Life" in Part 6). And I had to set limits with work (see "If It Can Be Done, It Must Be Done," also in Part 6) and accept the truth that I can't do everything.

I can finally say that I do have needs. I don't have supernatural powers. I'm not Wonder Woman. The supernatural thing about this is: I don't want to be.

The Sadness Cloud

Y EARS AGO, I sat in group therapy for my eating disorder and said, "I feel like a cloud of sadness is following me around today. It feels like drops of rain are coming out of an otherwise clear, blue sky."

I asked the other women, "Do you guys ever feel sad for no apparent reason?"

The overwhelming answer was yes, yes, and yes. In fact, every woman in group that day knew exactly what I was talking about. I was taken aback by their answers and felt like I was finally being let in on a big secret of life: *It's okay to feel sad.* I wondered why I hadn't received the sadness memo until then.

We live in a society that tells us we should be happy 24/7. If we're not happy, then a vitamin, a supplement, a pill, or perhaps the newest microwave oven will put a smile on our faces.

When I was a little kid in school, we were told that good kids didn't cry. So I didn't cry. The boys especially were singled out: "Boys don't cry." My sister-in-law, Destiny, is going against that grain and is teaching her sons that it is okay to be sad and to have feelings. It's okay to cry. My three-year-old nephew, Drew, already knows how to tell his mom, "I feel sad." Needless to say, Drew is years ahead of me in this area. It took me more than twenty years, plus group therapy, to be able to say those three little words, "I feel sad."

Throughout recovery, I became more and more connected with my true feelings. Instead of stuffing or starving away sorrow, I began to feel it. In this way, feeling sad was actually progress for me. Connecting with any of my real feelings was a good thing.

When I first gained an awareness of my feelings, I felt overwhelmed. I had rarely experienced my true emotions before, so everything seemed extraordinarily intense, and that frightened me. I actually thought there might be something wrong with me, but after working with Ann, I realized that my feelings were normal. I was normal.

When I felt sad, I began to say, "The sadness cloud is visiting me." Whether or not I could find a reason behind the sadness cloud, as a healthy adult, I needed to be accountable for taking care of myself.

First and foremost, I have learned that I don't have to do anything to make sadness (or any other feelings for that matter) go away. At the same time, I can do a lot of things to take care of myself while the sadness cloud is hanging over me. I can listen to my favorite song on repeat and sing. Or I can call someone I trust and talk about something unrelated (or related) to my sadness. Most of all, I can be gentle with myself and try not to have unrealistic expectations related to work or anything else.

These days, I try to remember that feeling sad is a part of life. I also respect my past history of depression and realize that I need to be ready to take serious action in the event that the sadness cloud becomes a hurricane. While I don't believe in simply popping a pill every time I feel down, I respect the fact that a psychiatrist and medication have helped me a lot in the past. So I keep an open mind about talking with my doctor and taking necessary medication in the future.

Notwithstanding my personal history of depression, I also remember that I have an even bigger history of turning something that is not really a big deal into a very big deal. So I try not to make the sadness cloud even bigger by feeling sad about feeling sad and hence become even sadder. I used to sabotage myself with negative thoughts like, "I will never be happy," or "I was just born to be sad." People talk a lot about the power of positive affirmations. Just think about the power of negative ones! When I found myself repeating those same old negative affirmations, it helped to separate from those thoughts and to connect with my heart. I have learned that I have a choice in whether or not I am pulled away from the present moment with negative, futuristic thinking. One new, positive affirmation that I find particularly helpful is "It's okay to be happy."

It's still okay to feel sad too. I know this is complicated. I often need the help of a therapist or good friend to sort through this stuff. Unlike Drew, I have not been naming and experiencing my feelings since I was three. I sometimes need a little more guidance than others. Even a three-year-old.

Real Action: Mood Chart

One of the most helpful tools in my life right now is not a hammer, screwdriver, or even my new iPhone. It is a mood chart that Ann encouraged me to keep in my journal. Each day, I note my mood by writing a number between 1 and 10 (1 = saddest, 10 = happiest). In addition to noting a number every day, I track my menstrual cycle and write any other important information like sleep patterns, medication changes, major life events, and so on.

Currently, I have about six months' worth of data that has helped me see patterns in my moods that I wouldn't have noticed otherwise. With my mood chart, I am better able to accept my moods, anticipate changes, and ride the ups and downs. (Similar to a weather forecaster, I am often able to track the sadness cloud.)

Try keeping a mood chart for yourself. You can use a scale from 1 to 10, 1 to 5, or something else entirely. The important thing is to create a system that you understand and works for you. Track your mood for a few months and see if you notice any patterns.

A Different Decision

IT IS A wonder that this book was ever written. I had wanted to write it for more than a year before I finally made the decision to do it. I said a lot of things during that time that sounded like decisions, things like the following:

I will write the book *after* I am finished researching the topic.
I will write the book *as long as* I am inspired.
I will write the book *unless* I am busy doing other things.

The problem was that research about life is never done, I don't wake up every day feeling inspired, and I'm always busy doing other things. Each "decision" had a threshold, as indicated by the words *after*, *as long as*, and *unless*. To write this book, I made a different decision: I will write the book. Period.

I learned about the importance of making a different decision from my work in recovery. Over the years, I had made countless decisions to recover from my eating disorder. I decided to recover when I told my boyfriend about my struggles and first asked for help. I decided to recover on the day I found out that my eating disorder had damaged my bones. I decided to recover after almost wrecking my car as a result of bingeing and purging.

I had decided to recover, but I was not recovered. I would experience months of Ed-free behavior, only to relapse again. Even when I wasn't bingeing, purging, or restricting, negative thoughts about food and my body consumed me. Any recovery I experienced was marginal at best. I wanted full freedom. Why couldn't I find it?

Looking back, I realize that my early decisions to divorce Ed looked a lot like my initial decisions to write this book. You might say they weren't really decisions at all:

I will stay in recovery *if* things stay the same in my life.
I will respect my body *as long as* I do not gain more weight.
I will stay on track with food *unless* I get the urge to binge.

Guess what? Things changed in my life, I gained weight, and I got the urge to binge. When I hit these thresholds, I went back to Ed. The thresholds meant that Ed was still an option in my life. His name was still scribbled somewhere on my list of Things I Do to Cope with Life. Sure, his name had moved from the top of that list to the bottom, which was an improvement, but it was still there. A different decision meant taking Ed off the list; he could not be an option. I had to recover.

Making a different decision was not easy. I didn't just wake up one day and say, "Gee, I think I will make a strong decision to recover today," and then presto, I was recovered. No, first I had to recognize that a strong desire is not the same as a strong decision. *Wanting* means something entirely different than *willing*. Wanting to recover is not the same as being willing to do whatever it takes to recover. I became willing to do whatever it took.

A strong decision acknowledges and respects the positive aspects of the eating disorder. Ed made me feel special and helped me relieve stress. I had to grieve letting go of these aspects of Ed and find other, healthier ways to accomplish the same things. (I have discovered that I'm special just by being me.)

A strong decision also involves drastic change and drastic action. For me, drastic change meant interrupting my relapses as soon as possible. A key to my personal recovery was stopping any and all purging behaviors following a binge. After I binged, I needed to do the next right thing, which meant not restricting, not overexercising, not purging in any way. Doing the next right thing meant eating the very next meal after a binge—today, not tomorrow. In the beginning, I felt like someone was ripping out my heart and soul every time I didn't purge. Sitting with food in my stomach felt unbearable. But it really wasn't unbearable; it was just unbelievably uncomfortable. Even so, I could not purge, no matter what—no thresholds.

To get through these difficult times and stay accountable for my actions, I had to connect with people on my support team. When I took care of myself like this, I often felt like a failure, like I was disappointing people. (Perhaps this had something to do with the fact that Ed was yelling, "You're a failure! You're disappointing people!" as loud as he possibly could.) But I was actually a success, and people were proud of me, even if I wasn't particularly proud of myself.

A strong decision ultimately meant a strong recovery. If I had never made a different decision to recover, I would not be recovered today. If I had never made a different decision to write this book, you wouldn't be reading it now. A different decision made all the difference.

Real Action: Your Different Decisions

Do you have any thresholds that are keeping you from a full recovery? Give it some thought, talk with someone on your support team, and complete the following statements:

I will stay on track with food *until* _____.
I will honor my body *as long as* _____.
I will exercise in a healthy way *unless* _____.

Now write three to five different decisions for your recovery.

The Hole

I'M SURE YOU know about the hole. It's that empty space inside that we all try to fill with something. Some of us will do almost anything to fill it. Or we will do almost anything to make it disappear so we don't have to fill it—or feel it—anymore.

It is that hole inside that you tried to fill with eating disordered behaviors. When that didn't work, you might have turned to drugs, alcohol, or both. Many people do—bouncing back and forth between an eating disorder and an addiction. Some of you turned to a man or a woman. Some turned to self-injury. No matter what you did, the hole was still there.

I used to be able to starve, purge, and binge the hole away temporarily. But eventually, my eating disorder stopped "working" altogether. I would still starve, purge, and binge, but the hole would still be there, only it was coupled with more pain.

Luckily, I was far enough along recovery road at that point to know that nothing external was going to fill the hole. Instead of acting out with other types of destructive behaviors (which I thought about but never did), I actually felt the hole, the pain beneath the eating disorder. It was raw, piercing, shaking, numbing, and immobilizing all at once—cutting to the bone. It was a deep space of loneliness, desperation, and hopelessness that seemed to penetrate my very core. Nothing had ever felt like this before. If this was recovery, I didn't want anything to do with it.

It turns out that the hole wasn't recovery; it just signified that I had more work to do. The hole is part of why I still needed therapy even though I was eating right and maintaining a healthy weight. (This was sometimes difficult for people in my life to understand.)

My friend Aaron, who is in recovery from alcoholism, says that the hole can only be filled with God. He compares it to filling the gas tank in your car. You can fill the tank with lemonade if you want. The tank will be full, but the car won't run. Gas is the only thing that will make your car go, and Aaron says that God is the only way to truly fill the hole inside of us.

To me, filling the hole with God meant filling it with all things spiritual. This involved not only connecting with God but also building relationships with people. (God often talks to me through other people.) It meant getting in touch with my heart, my feelings, and my passions. Music and nature are also spiritual experiences for me, because both connect me back to myself in a real, authentic way.

Part of filling up with God meant not being attached to results. If I believe that my life depends on this book becoming a *New York Times* bestseller, then I am too attached. When I recognize this kind of attachment, I have to step away and find peace in the moment.

My friend Nicole, who is in recovery from an eating disorder and an addiction, says, "To me, filling the hole with God meant I had to get out of myself and find a way to look at life as a gift and not a constant battle. I had to look at people as blessings and friends, not my competition or enemies."

I don't know if the hole ever actually goes away, but I do know that it doesn't have to go anywhere. The hole is not a personal deficit—it's just a part of being human. (We are whole even when we experience the hole.) As long as I am mindful, I can recognize the hole. I can notice any urges or compulsions that go along with it. I can make a decision not to let the hole interfere with my goals or my value system.

I can experience the hole and figure out what it's trying to tell me. Is it telling me that I need to grow in a new area? That I need to practice better self-care? That I need more balance in my life?

Today, I try not to pass judgment on the hole. I try to accept it and do the next right thing. For the most part, if I stay spiritually fit, the hole doesn't seem to have much power over me.

The concept of filling up with God might look different in your life. Maybe you use different words to define God and spirituality. Your job is to figure out what works for you.

I'm fairly certain that you won't fill your gas tank with lemonade. How will you choose to fill the hole inside?

Relapse Is Normal

RELAPSE IS A natural part of the recovery process. It's expected. For a long time, Ed used this very real information as ammunition against me. He would say, "Relapse is normal, Jenni. It's okay. Go ahead and just do what I say now, and I'll let you get back to that recovery stuff later."

In that moment, I would want the temporary relief Ed was offering more than recovery, so I would obey him, thinking, "Yes, relapse is expected. I'll stop relapsing sometime."

Sometime only happened when I stopped using the fact that relapse is normal as an excuse to relapse. It happened when I made a different decision to recover. It happened when I realized that I *did* have a choice in whether or not I continued to go back to Ed.

I used to believe that relapses were so natural and normal that they just sort of happened from out of the blue. I'd say, "I was doing great and then all of a sudden I felt like I was possessed by Ed. I had to binge."

Now I can see that I wasn't really doing great or I wouldn't have relapsed. I like to think of relapse as a process, rather than a specific event like bingeing, purging, or starving. For me, a binge never really began with the first compulsive bite, but much earlier. It began with my not taking care of myself in some other way.

I remember one particularly bad relapse that began with my being angry at a coworker. I didn't express my feelings to her, and over the period of a week, pent-up anger and resentment led to bingeing. At any point during that week, I could have made the decision to practice good self-care and avoid the relapse. But I didn't. Instead, I found myself staring at my refrigerator, ready to binge. As you can imagine, this is not the easiest time to make a good decision about whether or not to binge.

No, the best way for me to intervene on a relapse was always much earlier in the process. In the example of my coworker, the most effective way for me to interrupt the relapse would have been to experience my anger and to talk with her. If I had made that decision, I might never have found myself looking for answers in my refrigerator in the first place. The relapse didn't just happen because it was normal and expected. I had choices all along the way.

Of course, we have to learn how to intervene on a relapse at all points of the process—even if it is in the car at the drive-through window waiting for that food order. At this point, we can't just say, "Oh well, I didn't stop this binge earlier. I guess I'll have to go ahead and eat this food now. I'll start over with recovery tomorrow." We must always get back on track now, not later. I used to think it was impossible for me to stop eating in the middle of a binge. When my motto became "No excuses," I realized that I could, in fact, stop bingeing before Ed wanted me to. (You can, too.)

Yes, relapse is normal, but it doesn't always have to be. Do your best to learn something from each and every fall. Try not to fall in the same way twice, and ultimately you will fall less and less. Then relapse won't be normal for you anymore. Recovery will be normal. Recovered will be expected.

Important note: When I say "relapse," I am talking about anything from one episode of bingeing and purging (which some people might call a "lapse") to no longer following your recovery plan at all. I choose to use only the word "relapse" in this book because that is the term I used throughout my recovery to describe any setbacks. Along your journey, you and your treatment team might choose to distinguish between lapses and relapses. Like I always say, do what works.

3

THE DATING GAME

Exploring the World

No longer arm in arm with Ed, I was able to jump into the dating game. I'm not talking about getting to know lots of men; I'm talking about getting to know myself. My life was opened up to uncovering lost passions, exploring new activities, and adopting beliefs that coincided with my true thoughts and desires. My outlook on life and my definition of happiness changed. As I moved closer to my true identity, Ed seemed further and further away. Exploring the world and finding out who I am has been both exciting and challenging. Dating can be scary, so Part 3 is here to help.

Finding Me (for the First Time)

RECOVERY FROM MY eating disorder not only meant getting rid of Ed, but more importantly, it meant getting Jenni back. It meant finding out who I am, what I like to do, and what I really believe. Recovery was not necessarily about building Jenni, but rather about uncovering a Jenni who had always been there but I never knew. Ed had never wanted me to find her and had, in fact, kept her hidden. My eating disorder had become my identity. Ira Sacker, M.D., speaks about the importance of breaking free from the eating disorder identity in his book, *Regaining Yourself.*

I remember telling my therapy group once about an awakening I'd had. No, not the key to perpetual happiness or anything like that. I had figured out my favorite color. In group, I said, "My favorite color is pink, and I think it always has been. The funny thing is that I don't own many pink things." So I began to surround myself with the color pink, which made me smile. (Don't worry, my home doesn't look like it's coated with Pepto-Bismol.)

Similar to discovering my favorite color, I realized that I love nature and that my life didn't reflect this either. I rarely, if ever, did anything outside. I checked my mailbox and took out the trash, but that was about it for my outdoor activities. Getting healthy meant making changes in my life to reflect who I am. First, under the advice of my treatment team, I began to take short walks in my neighborhood. I enjoyed looking at the trees, especially the beautiful fall colors in Tennessee. As I became healthier, I began to hike with friends at a nearby state park. Recently, I have taken many trips to Alaska just to be out in the middle of nature; I have been ice climbing, snowshoeing, and cross-country skiing. There aren't many snow sports where I live in Nashville, but there is a lot of mountain biking.

After thinking about it for months, I finally bought a mountain bike. Of course, I wanted a pink bike but had to settle for a blue one with pink accessories.

Finding my true self didn't just include figuring out my favorite color or that I loved nature, although these were good places to start. I also became more in tune with my beliefs and values. I first learned that Ed and I had different values. While he thought that being thin was more important than my family, friends, or anything else, I intellectually knew that wasn't true. Ed's values were insane and irrational. I slowly connected more and more with my true values. Even more slowly, I began to align my actions with those values.

Later in recovery, I realized that I lived by many insane, irrational beliefs not related to food and weight at all. As a therapy assignment, I once made a list (unrelated to eating disordered behaviors) in my journal titled "Insane, Irrational Beliefs that I Live By." Here is one belief from that list: *If I date someone, I will always lose my dreams and be miserable.*

I learned that a definitive statement like this (made clear by the word *always*) is a sign that a belief might be irrational. Another sign is when the belief only applies to me, which was the case here. You could be in a relationship and be fine, but not me. In therapy, I learned to counteract my insane beliefs with rational and reasonable statements based on the same information. For instance, the aforementioned belief became *It is possible for people to lose their dreams and be miserable by giving their power away to another person.*

This step helped me to depersonalize the belief, allowing me to make room for a new, healthy belief. In this instance, my new belief became *If I keep my power in a dating relationship, another person can't control my dreams and feelings.*

This belief is reasonable and could actually help me to not give my power away to another person in a dating relationship. The original belief just kept me out of relationships completely, which actually gave all of my power away—by taking away the freedom of choice. Even though much of my prerecovered belief system was, in fact, irrational, I resisted changing something I had become so invested in. I began to change only when I fully accepted that I would never be happy living within the constraints of such beliefs. Therapy and life experience were key to helping me connect with new, healthy beliefs (my true beliefs). I learn more about what I believe every day.

Despite Ed's best efforts, I have finally found *me* for the first time. Me changes as I grow. Uncovering pieces of myself is an exciting journey, one that I don't expect to end as long as I am walking around on the planet.

Real Action: Finding You

Instead of putting all your focus on getting rid of Ed, start thinking about getting to know yourself. That's what recovery is all about anyway.

Get in touch with your heart and answer the following questions. If you're like me, in the beginning, you might find that you know more about who you are *not* than who you are. If so, then start there. If you don't know your favorite color (the first question here), list colors that you know are not your favorites.

1. What is your favorite color? _____
2. What outdoor activities do you enjoy? _____
3. What indoor activities do you enjoy? _____

Now, here's the fun part! Make sure your life reflects your answers in some way. If you listed playing board games as an enjoyable indoor activity, spend more time doing that. On the other hand, if you listed playing board games as something you don't enjoy, pass on the next invite to play Trivial Pursuit.

Why Me?

TODAY WAS EITHER a really bad day or a really good day. Let me explain.

I was finishing up a section in this book when I decided to take a quick power nap. While I was napping, my Mac decided to go to sleep too. The difference between my computer and me is that I woke up. It didn't.

After going to the Mac Store and talking with four Geniuses, the guys at Mac who can fix everything, I was told they couldn't fix this. My hard drive, which contained many years' worth of work on this book, was dead. Really bad news!

Tears fell down my face until one of the Geniuses said that the backup program I had installed on my computer only two days earlier had been working correctly, which meant that my data would be okay. Really good news! I left my computer at the store, so they could install a new hard drive.

I headed home in my car and let out a big sigh of relief—just before a big pickup truck rear-ended me. My sigh of relief was replaced by a police officer, two banged-up vehicles, a scared young man (the driver of the truck who ran into me), and one mad girlfriend (the owner of the truck). As I thought about the hassle of getting my car and computer fixed, I wondered why both of these things had to crash in the same day. A bit of self-pity crept in as I asked, "Why me?"

In the past, I was a perpetual victim; how I was doing in any given moment depended on what happened to me. Today I do my best to avoid this kind of "victim thinking." Instead, how I am doing is determined by how I respond to what happens to me. "Why me?" has become a springboard for the question "Why not me?" We all get bumped in life. Why should I be the exception?

The cool thing is that I know how to handle bumps now without spiraling out of control. (For those of you who read *Life Without Ed*, you know that a fender bender was once a reason to binge. I'm glad those days are over.)

The really good news about the car accident is that no one was physically injured. If anything, I was actually helped by getting yet another chance to practice not being a victim and by gaining a new perspective on my busy, book-writing life. The car crash opened my eyes—yet again—to just how fragile life is. In the blink of an eye, someone could have been killed. A couple of hours earlier, I had been in tears because my life's work might have vanished from my computer. Losing data is nothing compared to losing my life.

As I write this tonight, I feel a sore throat coming on. I probably picked up a cold that a couple of my friends have been battling. That's the bad news. The good news is twofold. First, I actually have true friends from whom I pick up illnesses these days. Second, one of my other friends is in medical school, and she is coming over to help me out. She mentioned something about gargling salt water.

All in all, my computer crashed, my car got wrecked, my throat hurts, and now I get to gargle salt water. Today has been a really good day. Why me?

Guitar: Take Two

WHAT DO YOU get when you add recovery to a guitar? You get a guitar player.

When I first tried to learn how to play the guitar, I found the experience frustrating and painful. I ultimately shoved the guitar into the back of my closet and gave up. Today my guitar is out of the closet, and learning to play is a completely different experience.

The difference is simply that I am recovered. When I tried to learn how to play ten years ago, I was at the height of my battle with Ed. Back then, the guitar felt like a foreign object that was invading my space—as most things did with Ed around. Now I love feeling the guitar next to me. I can actually feel the vibrations resonate throughout my body. I never felt them back then, because I was so disconnected from my body. The guitar is no longer threatening; instead, it is a part of me. We are connected.

I am physically stronger now as well. Pressing down the strings used to seem nearly impossible. Now the muscles in my fingers are strong enough to hold down the strings with no problem at all. I also have more energy in general and can focus clearly. There is no struggle. I used to feel like the guitar was fighting me; now I feel like we are working together. (When I was struggling with my eating disorder, I often felt like I was under attack, if not by my guitar, then by someone or something else.)

I remember dreading going to my guitar lessons, because I thought I had to perform perfectly. I look forward to my lessons these days, and I don't worry about doing anything perfectly. I actually had a lesson today, and I completely forgot about a homework assignment that my teacher, Ellen Britton, had given me. I laughed and said that I'd forgotten. Ellen just smiled, and we had a great lesson. She constantly reminds me of my progress as a guitar player, and I accept her positive feedback without fighting it. With Ed, I always pushed away the good and only heard the bad. Today, I let the good in.

When I first tried to learn the guitar, I remember thinking in an all-or-none kind of way that I was not a real guitar player, that I would be one only when I could stand up in front of a large audience and play complicated songs. Today, I can only play a handful of songs, including "Amazing Grace" and "Rudolph the Red-Nosed Reindeer," and my audience is usually just my three-year-old nephew. I still call myself a real guitar player, and my nephew thinks I'm a rock star. It is all about perspective. Back then, I remember thinking, "Why should I even bother to learn how to play the guitar? I will be too old by the time I can play well. It will take at least ten years."

It's ten years later, and I can see now that I am not too old for anything. In fact, I wish I hadn't stopped playing back then, because I would be playing with ease by now. Rather than losing any more time to Ed or negative thinking, I'm just going to keep on playing. Take two with my guitar has been a fun and exciting experience. Take two with my life has been worlds better than that! Being recovered brings a new joy to everything I do. Are *you* ready for take two?

Jenni Deserves a Kitchen Table

I AM WRITING MUCH of this book sitting at my desk in my office. Because I'm single and living in a small place, my office is actually my dining room, and my desk is my kitchen table covered by file organizers, pens, notepads, and, of course, my laptop.

While I am writing about finding my own identity apart from an eating disorder, my kitchen table has lost its identity. I find it a little ironic that I can't even eat here because it is covered up with my work about learning how to eat again. (Note: I am still eating, just not at my kitchen table.)

In addition to this table, my entire home seems to be covered with eating disorder material. My living room actually looks like a resource center with books, brochures, and even Love Your Body lotion giveaways. When friends drop by, I can offer them not only a cup of coffee and something to eat but also body lotion and a *How to Help a Friend with an Eating Disorder* pamphlet. I admit that this setup is not an ideal living environment. I need to find a way to separate my work from my home.

Along with that, I deserve to live in a space that is clutter free. The eating disorder material that covers my home is not always well organized. I have recovered from my eating disorder, and now I need to recover from clutter and disorganization.

I explained my home environment, including the kitchen table situation, to my friend Rich, and I gave him many excuses. I said, "I haven't had a kitchen table in years. In fact, my last three apartments were so small that none of them even had a dining room, much less a place to fit a kitchen table. I've gotten used to eating at my coffee table."

Rich, who knows me well, interrupted and simply said, "Jenni deserves a kitchen table." He continued by saying that I deserve to have a home that supports healthy living, a place that helps me feel peaceful and grounded.

Yes, I do! Part of being recovered means that my tolerance for stuff that I used to just live with has gone down a lot. I used to be content with my work taking over my entire house. As someone who never stopped working, I actually found it convenient to see my work all over the place. Needless to say, I do not find it convenient anymore. I find it distracting.

I have worked very hard to recover from an eating disorder, and now I want to live in a place that reflects my newfound inner peace. I need to make changes in my home and will start by reclaiming my kitchen table.

As I wrote that last sentence, excuses instantly poured into my head as to why getting my table back will be impossible. But I know that if I can recover from an eating disorder, I can surely solve a simple furniture problem. After recovering from an eating disorder, most of my "problems" end up not being problems at all.

I'm going to leave you right now, reclaim my kitchen table, and get back with you when I'm done.

DONE. IT TOOK last night and this morning, but I figured it out. I gave away some things, reorganized my books, and my kitchen table is back. It is again a kitchen table. My dining room is a dining room. The delineation between my work and my home is notably better, and there is even less clutter. I feel better; my mind is less cluttered.

My friend was right. I do deserve a kitchen table. I deserve to live in a peaceful environment. And so do you!

Real Action: What Do You Deserve?

Is your living space conducive to living a recovered life? Don't feel bad if it isn't; you know my story. What is one thing that you can do to your home right now to help you feel more centered? Sort through a pile of paper, take out the trash, or just light a candle?

If you lean toward compulsivity in the home department (and tend to keep your home immaculately clean and organized), making a change for the better might actually mean throwing some clothes on the floor. I always tended to keep my home messy (the "if it can't be perfect, it might as well be a disaster" attitude), so progress for me would have been picking up some of the clothes.

It doesn't matter if your home is an apartment, dorm room, house, treatment center, or something else. It is still your home. Make a change for the better!

I Will Be Happy When . . .

I will be happy when I'm rail thin. *I wasn't.*
I will be happy when I'm at a healthy weight and no longer
act out in eating disordered behaviors. *Nope.*
I will be happy when I get engaged to Mark. *That didn't
work.*
I will be happy when I break my engagement with Mark.
Wrong again.
I will be happy when I quit my job waiting tables and work
full-time as a writer. *You guessed it, not happy.*

What is the common denominator in all of these situations?
Me.

I changed my job, but not myself. I left Mark, but I was still
with me. I even changed my body, but I was the same person on
the inside. I changed external things from my body to my relationship to my job and more, but the internal stuff stayed the
same. Looking to the external world to fix an internal problem
didn't work. The truth is that if you take care of the internal, the
external takes care of itself.

Sure, my skinny size, Mark, and my new job all brought about
short-lived, immediate highs and fleeting moments of excitement,
but they did not bring about genuine happiness. In fact, each one
only brought with it the fear that I might lose it again. Being thin
created intense anxiety that I wouldn't be able to maintain that
weight for life, and I couldn't. The high of dating Mark brought
about the fear of losing him, which I did. With the new lifestyle
as a full-time writer came the fear that I wouldn't be able to make
a living at it forever. (We'll see how long this one lasts.)

I have no idea how long you will keep reading my books and listening to what I have to say. I can't control that. Instead of fearing it, I try to accept that I can lose anything external at any time and focus on the fact that the only thing I will always have is myself. I might not always have my fingers and toes, but my heart will always be intact. Whether or not I connect with it is up to me.

To focus inwardly, I have had to change my definition of happiness. Happiness is not being thin, having a successful career, or dating the perfect guy. Happiness comes from doing the next real and right thing in the here and now. In other words, I am happy when I take the information I have in each moment and live honestly. Happiness is a sense of peace and serenity that lives within me despite what is going on outside of me. Even in what society deems as the worst situations, I'm told that we can still feel this inner peace. My friend Aaron often reminds me that the prisoner on death row can be happy while the businessman in the big, corner office can be miserable. It took a while, but I finally believe him.

I also finally believe that I just need to be rather than do, to be real and connect with my breath in each moment. I need to let my heart guide me rather than follow my mind and all of its thoughts. Connecting with my heart is my connection to God. It is my connection to happiness.

Today I sense inner serenity more than ever before. I especially feel it when I am in nature, listening to music, or meditating. My challenge is to keep this inner connectedness when I have a disagreement with my cell phone company or am stuck in a bumper-to-bumper traffic jam. In those moments, instead of saying I will be happy when my cell phone company gives in and when I get out of the traffic jam, I need to say that I will be happy right now. I can choose to be happy now.

Living in the Moment?

*T*HE ONLY MOMENT *we have is right now.* Blah, blah, blah. Whatever. Yeah, right. I used to hate reading sentences like that!

As a type A, perfectionistic workaholic, I believed that authors like Eckhart Tolle who emphasized living in the present moment just wanted me to lie around all day on my couch meditating and being lazy. I thought, "What better way for Tolle and those other authors to ensure the success of their books than to convince writers like me to sit around doing nothing."

I thought, "I won't be fooled," and continued on with avoiding the present as much as possible. I continued worrying about the past and the future—wondering "what if this" and "what if that." While I was thinking about what if, I was nowhere near what is, nowhere near now.

But I kept gravitating toward Tolle's book, *The Power of Now.* I would read it over and over only to read it yet again. Gradually, I began to believe that his message actually might be something I could apply in my life.

Other people I know, including Ann, kept talking about living in the moment as well. In therapy sessions, Ann would say, "Be still and just go inside. Breathe. Listen to what your heart is telling you right now." I would get frustrated, thinking, "I'm paying a lot of money to talk with you, not to sit here on your couch in complete silence." I thought I had figured Ann out too. If she just told her clients to be quiet and still, then she didn't have to do any work. She didn't even have to speak. Smart lady.

Through experimentation of my own (aka pain), I have discovered that Tolle, Ann, and the others were not looking out for themselves but were actually trying to share important information with me. Tolle wasn't trying to stave off competition from another writer, and Ann wasn't trying to get me to do her job for her: I had to learn to be quiet with myself and accept the present moment.

In my life today, I do my best to stay in the present. I do this in various ways, including giving myself quiet time each morning and evening, and spending time outside in nature. Sometimes I take a gentle yoga class. Ann recently challenged me to keep some awareness of my breath throughout my daily activities. This is difficult for me, so I have actually placed Post-it notes throughout my home with the word *Now* written on them with a black marker. Each time I see one of these notes, I breathe and try to focus on the present. When I do this, I find peace. I am happy.

Looking back, I can see that Ed was great at pulling me away from the present with bingeing, purging, and restricting; with worrying about the weight I had already gained and the weight I might still have to lose. Since he was all about avoiding the present, it is no surprise to me that in my life after Ed, living in the moment is still a challenge. I have not had a lot of practice with it yet, but I have confidence that I will continue to be more present with each and every day. I will start right now. After all, like I said at the beginning: the only moment we have *is* right now.

Real Action: Worry Journal

Worrying kept me in my eating disorder and out of the present moment. The first step to battling my hyperactive worry muscle was awareness. During my therapy work, I actually kept track of the amount of time I wasted on worrying in a "worry journal." Throughout the week, I listed everything I worried about. I recorded the date and time that I began to worry about each issue and then recorded the date and time when each issue was resolved.

I calculated the amount of time I had wasted worrying and recorded that in my worry journal as well. I wasted hours and hours of precious time that could have been devoted to living my life. Here are a couple of excerpts from my journal:

> **Wednesday, 2 P.M.:** *Janet is mad at me. She has not returned my phone call yet.*
> **Thursday, 3 P.M.:** *Janet called me back. She was not mad, just busy.*
> **Time wasted worrying:** *25 hours*
> **Monday, 9 A.M.:** *I will never complete the project on time. I will get fired.*
> **Thursday, 8 A.M.:** *I finished the project right on time. I wasn't fired.*
> **Time wasted worrying:** *71 hours*

Most of what I worried about turned out fine or really didn't matter anyway. If something that I worried about did come true and did actually matter, I realized that I could have just waited to worry about it until it happened. Why waste time and energy worrying about the same thing twice? More important, why worry at all?

Does worrying keep you out of the present moment? Keep track of wasted time in your own worry journal. Then promise to make a change. Put energy into what you can change; don't worry about the rest. This is a helpful application of the Serenity Prayer (see "God Hates Me?" in Part 2).

Live in the Solution

CAN YOU MAKE a mountain out of a molehill? I used to be an expert at it. Heck, I could make a mountain out of anything. If you gave me a grain of sand, a speck of dust, or even an empty coffee can, I could make a mountain. I was an expert problem finder.

I was especially talented at creating problems out of things that really weren't problems at all, out of good things, out of the best of circumstances. If I had won a million dollars in the lottery, I would have complained about paying taxes on it. If someone had given me a free trip to Hawaii, I would have agonized over planning the trip. If one of my dreams came true, I would think, "It won't be long before I lose this."

During treatment for my eating disorder, my problem-finding abilities came to the forefront. My treatment team noticed that I gave Ed more airtime than Jenni. In other words, I spent more time reporting what Ed was saying than talking about what I was saying. As time went by, members of the team began to say, "I know what Ed says. I want to know what Jenni says." They wanted me to live in the solution instead of the problem. I thought they were crazy.

Couldn't they see that my eating disorder was ruining my life? Didn't they know that food was my biggest problem?

Apparently not, because they kept telling me, "Food is not your problem; it's your solution." Ha, ha, ha! I thought they were very clever. (Notice the sarcasm here. I still thought these people were crazy.)

I discovered they weren't crazy, but they were right. Food was, in fact, my solution. It wasn't a good one, but it was a solution. Restricting food, eating too much food, and purging food was my solution to both real and make-believe problems. I needed to find other solutions—ones that really worked and were conducive to healthy living. I needed to be a solution finder instead of a problem finder.

Interestingly enough, I also needed to focus on being a *solution finder* rather than a *problem solver*. Focusing on solving a problem often kept me in the problem, rooting around in the dirt, looking for a way out; focusing on finding solutions catapulted me out of the problem and forced me to look at it from a new perspective. This small shift in focus made a big difference in my life. Oftentimes, especially during my recovery, I didn't need to think about everything I was doing wrong; instead, I needed to focus more on what I was doing right—and then do more of the right stuff. I needed to live more in the solution.

I still catch myself making a mountain out of a molehill (or out of anything at all) from time to time. When this happens, I do my best to walk away from the mountain and head toward the solution. That's where I want to live these days.

Where do you live? Where do you want to live?

Real Action: Where Do You Live?

Take some time to write answers to the two questions at the end of this section. Here's one more: What is one thing you can do today to live in the solution?

Alaska in Tennessee

WHEN I WAS returning home from a trip the other day—in a plane about to land at the airport—I looked out the window and thought, "Wow! I live in Nashville." As a little kid, I had always loved country music and had dreamed about living here someday. When I first moved to the city about ten years ago, I often thought the same thing: "Wow! I live in Nashville." I remember driving around town with my eyes wide, trying to take everything in.

Over the years, as I battled my eating disorder and fought hard to recover, any excitement I'd once had for living in the city disappeared in a cloud of dust. Even when I stopped experiencing eating disordered behaviors, I felt bad most of the time, and many times, I actually blamed my problems on Nashville. I thought, "I need to move away from here. Then I will feel better." That would have been a geographical cure for an internal problem, and that doesn't work.

So I stayed put, and slowly, little by little, my recovered life has brought back that original excitement that I had for living in Nashville (and for life in general). Strangely, my love for Tennessee started coming back when I began to visit Alaska. In that beautiful state, I could get lost in nature—hiking, ice fishing, glacier watching, and more. In Alaska, my cell phone and Internet connection also didn't work too well, so I could find peace from gadgets that I never had back home. Even when my phone was working, people from the Lower 48 tended not to call me, mistakenly believing that America's last frontier didn't have electricity or other modern conveniences.

I once said to a friend who lives in Anchorage, "I love Alaska. There are so many things to do. And it's so peaceful."

He replied, "There are a lot of things to do where you live. It could be peaceful there too."

"Yes," I thought to myself. "He's right."

When I got back to Nashville from that particular trip, I began to explore my own city. Tennessee is a beautiful state with lots of outdoor activities—just like Alaska. I joined an outdoor adventure group and also found some people to go mountain biking with on the many trails scattered throughout the area. I realized that a fun group of people my age played volleyball in a park near my house every Tuesday night in the summer. I had a blast with these people last summer. If I had just been paying more attention to life (and less attention to my problems), I could have had a blast with them the summer before and maybe the one before that too. In addition to all of these great outdoor activities, Nashville is also Music City, USA—a town with so much talent and creativity that you can hear great music almost any time of the day, every day of the week. As an artist myself, I know that the best studios and songwriters are right at my doorstep.

I have even discovered how to get hours of uninterrupted time in Nashville coffee shops. All I have to do is turn off my cell phone and disconnect from the Internet. Yes, this is possible! I used to think I had to "earn" rest or space and that I had to go on vacation—in Alaska—to get it. Even though it is almost socially unacceptable these days to be out of touch, I sometimes am. For my personal well-being, it's necessary.

I used to travel to Alaska to find peace and have fun. I still love Alaska, and I will keep visiting, but it's nice to know that I don't have to travel 4,043.42 miles (according to Yahoo! Maps) to find peace and have fun. I have created my own Alaska right here in Tennessee. Ed kept me from seeing the world around me, but now my new, recovered eyes are wide open. I love what I see.

Do you need a little Alaska? You don't have to hop on a plane. You just need to keep working to make your divorce from Ed final, and while you're doing that, be a tourist in your own town. Get excited about the world around you. Get excited about your life!

What You See Is What You Get

"YOU SEEM REALLY happy," my friend Wynde said to me the other day. "Your shoulders are relaxed, and you just look calm and peaceful."

She did *not* say, "You smile more than anyone I know," which is what people used to tell me as I smiled constantly to hide the pain I felt on the inside. No, Wynde said that I seemed happy, because I am happy. I didn't even have to smile.

Recently, another friend, Rob, said, "You look different these days. You seem more relaxed and less rigid. You seem more comfortable in your body." He did *not* say that I am the thinnest person he has ever known. These days, I would much rather hear that I look comfortable in my body, because I finally am.

And yet another friend, Chris, said, "You seem more confident." He did *not* say that I have achieved more accolades than everyone else. He said that I seem more confident in who I am as a person. I feel that way too.

What you see is what you get. My outside finally matches my inside. For so much of my life, my outside (what you saw) was incongruent with my inside (what I felt). I was a master actress, and I fooled everyone. My mom even called me the other day after reading parts of this book and said, "I never knew you felt all of those things growing up. We always thought you were so happy and well adjusted. It's like you were leading two different lives." I was, in fact, leading two lives, and I didn't even realize it myself. Ed had fooled me.

One of Ed's biggest lies to me was that he could deliver happiness—or if not happiness, at least some relief—directly to my door. It turned out that he could deliver pizza, but never happiness. One of the reasons I stayed with him for so long was that I kept buying into this particular lie. He had convinced me that as long as my body was thin, I would feel good on the inside. Being thin did give me short-lived bursts of self-esteem and confidence, but they faded away almost as quickly as they came. Back then, people regularly told me things ranging from "You have the perfect body," to "You're too skinny, look horrible, and need to gain weight." I took both remarks as compliments, and I would feel good on the inside—again, for a little while. In the long run, the more I fought to be thin, the more miserable I became. When I reached my lowest weight and was still unhappy, I finally began to accept that Ed was lying to me. Looking good (or what Ed said was good) on the outside didn't mean that I was doing well on the inside.

Although I didn't realize it at the time, much of my work in recovery, including overcoming codependency, feeling my feelings, and nurturing my body, was about becoming a more congruent person. I used to take care of others without taking care of myself. I used to reject inner feelings of sadness and smile on the outside. I used to starve in front of others and then binge in secret. Not anymore.

Wynde, Rob, and Chris gave me some of the best compliments I have ever received. They told me that I am congruent. I would much rather hear that than some comment about the size of my body.

Today people finally see the real me, inside and out.

Real Action: Inside/Outside Box

Find an empty box (a shoe box will work) and decorate the inside of it to show how you feel on the inside. Decorate the outside to show how other people see you. Get creative: use old fabric, clippings from newspapers and magazines, magic markers and crayons, and anything else that will help you express yourself safely. You might want to talk with your therapist and do this project in a session.

When I made my first inside/outside box in therapy, the inside was dark and dreary, while the outside was brightly colored. The box clearly showed that my inside did not match my outside. What does your box tell you?

4

GETTING ENGAGED

Relationships and More

I'm engaged! Not to a man. I'm engaged in healthy relationships that lift me up and empower me. When Ed and I were together, my tolerance for being in unhealthy (even downright abusive) relationships was high. Ed and I were dysfunctional, and so were many other relationships in my life. Today I fill my life with satisfying, loving relationships—from my friends and family to work colleagues to the people I choose to date. To my surprise, the more I work on my relationships, the more I learn about myself. If you want to get engaged too (without the fancy diamond ring), then turn the page and read Part 4.

Owning My Own Life

I'M FORGETTING TO breathe. I have a knot in my stomach. My limbs are going weak. I just took one more step toward truly owning my own life. I took some power back emotionally, and now I feel weak physically.

I just set a boundary with a work colleague, Megan, as a result of something Ann asked me in a therapy session today: "How many people on this planet are you going to let have authority over you?"

Yikes! Those words really hit home. The last time I looked at my birth certificate, it said Jennifer Lynn Schaefer. That is my name. I think that means that I'm the owner of my life. Despite lots of progress in this area, I am still handing my power over to other people—often in the name of codependency. Owning my own life means that I do not have to please people. Instead, I want to be polite and respectful to others while setting and protecting my own boundaries.

Owning my life also means that I maintain healthy limits rather than simply building brick walls. I used to be great at wall building. When it came to dating, my brick wall sounded something like this: I don't need a man, and I won't date. Not dating in order to control my dating life was only the illusion of control. Truly owning my life meant building boundaries that are flexible and give me room to grow—in my own time.

After my therapy session today, I called Megan and started setting some ground rules, including changing some plans related to our lunch meeting tomorrow. I only made a slight change, but it was important to me.

I took my power back, and that is when this weak feeling began. Ironically, this physically weak feeling signifies that I'm actually getting stronger. I know from my past that I will ultimately feel strong if I just sit with the feeling and experience it. I also know that with enough practice, setting boundaries and owning my own life will become natural and feel good. I won't always feel bad immediately after setting limits.

So here I am, sitting with the feeling. I'm not enjoying it. Sitting here feeling bad is certainly not what I want to be doing right now. But I'm not even thinking about turning to eating disordered behaviors to deal with how I feel. In fact, I wouldn't even have thought about Ed except for the fact that I'm writing this piece about life after an eating disorder.

Today I can take care of myself, feel uncomfortable, and do things that are difficult to do without thinking about Ed. This is huge progress for me, because in the past I actually used Ed to set boundaries. Years ago, instead of calling Megan and being honest with her, I would have simply binged. Then I would have canceled tomorrow's lunch meeting altogether. (That looks a lot more like a wall than a boundary, huh?)

Today I didn't have to binge, and I didn't have to cancel anything. Instead of using Ed, I used my voice to set a strong boundary on my own. I am Jennifer Lynn Schaefer, the owner of my life.

Whose name is on *your* birth certificate?

Real Action: Owning Your Own Life

When I was twenty-seven, one of my therapy assignments involved making two lists: how I had owned my life up to that point and how I hadn't. Here are a few examples from my lists:

How I Have *Not* Owned My Life Up to Age Twenty-Seven

- I let my ex-boyfriend dictate our relationship.
- I made many big decisions just to make other people happy.
- I have not made my own decisions related to spirituality.

How I *Have* Owned My Life Up to Age Twenty-Seven

- I broke up with my boyfriend.
- I fought back against Ed.
- I moved to Nashville on my own.

Try making your own lists. Depending on your age, your lists might be similar to or completely different from mine. It's your life, so write what is true for you—whether you are fifteen, thirty, or sixty.

Seven-Person Couch

M
Y FRIEND DAVE just bought and fixed up an amazing house. During the remodeling process, he said he wanted to make his home warm and welcoming, a good place to have get-togethers with friends. He moved in last weekend and has already had a couple of small gatherings. Last night, we fit seven people on his couch to watch a movie. I left Dave's house and realized how different my life and mind-set toward life are today.

When Ed and I first moved to Nashville ten years ago, I dreaded the idea of having people over to my home. In fact, I didn't own a couch or furniture for guests to sit on. There was no space for people in my home, but even more important, there was no room for them in my heart. The perceived demands of relationships overwhelmed me. Ed had convinced me that I was better off alone, that people would just take time away from my work. And, of course, they would want me to eat with them at lunches, dinners, parties, and so on. I avoided going out to social events at all costs, and I didn't have get-togethers in my own home.

The last thing I wanted was for people to hang out at my house having fun and infecting my territory with chips and dip and other party foods. The last thing I wanted was a seven-person couch. It seemed to me that a couch would simply attract people. (If you buy it, they will come.) Similar to my attitude toward food, I had anorexic tendencies toward people: "I don't need food, and I don't need them." Was I ever wrong!

In the past, hanging out with friends was something I did out of obligation. I knew I had to do something with friends every once in a while to keep them in my life. (I guess something deep inside me knew that I did need people.) I did the bare minimum required to hold the title of "friend." I learned that this is a good way to keep the title, but not a good way to keep a friendship. I never initiated get-togethers with anyone, but I would occasionally say yes to them.

It wasn't that I didn't like my friends or have fun with them. In fact, it was quite the opposite. I had so much fun that being around my friends made me feel unbearably guilty. I felt guilty for having fun instead of working and being productive. (Back then, I thought the only way to be productive was to work. I was wrong about that one too.) My friends were great, and that made me feel bad. Truly accepting their love and concern caused me to feel so anxious and uncomfortable that I blocked it out as best I could.

In the recovery process, I slowly learned to let people into my life on a whole new level. The women in my therapy group were the first ones I let in. I remember them inviting me out for coffee after group each week, and I remember saying no week after week. They kept asking, and I finally said yes. The first few times I went out with them, I felt—you guessed it—guilty. This was positive guilt, which I talked about in *Life Without Ed*, the kind of guilt that you feel when you are making progress and breaking rules that need to be broken. I also felt anxious, uncomfortable, and just plain bad. Sometimes feeling bad in recovery means that you're actually doing well.

After years of letting go little by little, I no longer feel guilty for spending time with friends. I actually look forward to that time and feel incredibly grateful for the wonderful people in my life. I have realized that I need friends, just like I need food. Isolation is not an option for me anymore.

My current home reflects this growth. I finally own a couch, and people sit on it often. But it was not the couch that attracted people; it was me. My couch won't hold seven like Dave's, but my heart will hold more. And that is what really matters.

Thirty-Two-Year-Old Adolescent

"You are in your adolescence and just now starting to date," Ann explained in a recent therapy session.

Which makes me a thirty-two-year-old adolescent! That may sound strange to you, but it feels completely accurate to me. I have always felt years behind people my age in the area of dating and sexuality. Clinicians have told me that our emotional development is arrested at the age that an eating disorder takes control of our lives. After we recover, we pick up emotionally where we left off at that age. So when it comes to dating, I feel like a teenager trapped in a thirty-two-year-old's body. I haven't had much experience dating, so I have a difficult time with relationships. I struggle to make sense of them.

I dated a little in high school—two proms and the occasional dinner and a movie. But Ed played a role in all of those events. Then, in college, Ed and I were so tight that he only let me go out with one guy two times throughout my entire four years. Ed went with me on those two dates as well. And he joined me on attempts I made at dating throughout my twenties. These attempts were few and far between due to two very long periods of jadedness during which I claimed to hate men. These periods directly followed the only two long-term relationships that I have had. I wasn't developmentally ready to be in those relationships, much less to handle the breakups in a healthy manner, without becoming extremely cynical and resentful.

Ed completely consumed my first relationship at age twenty-two. The other one, my relationship with Mark, was something I just jumped into without truly dating (getting to know someone slowly over time) beforehand. And Ed made brief appearances in that relationship too.

I am finally healthy and recovered, so I'm finally dating—for real this time. I'm also fully present on dates—just me without Ed. I am finding that as dysfunctional as my relationship with Ed was, at least dating him felt familiar and reliable. He was a predictable little weasel I could count on to inevitably make me feel horrible. Real people are not as predictable. Some guys do their best to treat me with kindness and genuine respect, which feels weird, and others don't treat me so well, which feels more like being with Ed. My challenge has been to stay with the nice guys and the weird feelings. When it comes to personal growth, weird is good. It means I'm moving into new and exciting territory; I'm making progress.

With Ann's help, I am learning that dating is fun, messy, and hard work. She says, "This is a developmental phase that will serve you well." I'm excited about exploring this adolescent phase of my adult life. Not many adults have a good excuse to act like a teenager!

No matter how old you are—clock time or developmental time—I hope you are excited about your life too. I hope you appreciate your current experience for what it's worth, for what you're learning. If your experience is anything like mine, you are probably finding out that you are behind in certain areas of life due to your eating disorder, but you are light-years ahead in other areas. For instance, I have known adults in recovery who didn't know the first thing about dating or even about balancing a checkbook, but they knew a lot more than the average person about family dynamics and spirituality (thanks to work in recovery).

I used to think that I was a freak of nature because I wasn't as experienced in dating as other thirty-somethings. I now understand that life is a process and I'm right where I'm supposed to be. My guess is that you are too.

(I have to confess that although I have made lots of progress in the dating arena, I am still very jaded about one thing: I would be hard-pressed to date a guy named Ed!)

Real Action: What Do You Want in a Relationship?

I recently found two lists I had created in my journal years ago, prior to meeting Mark. Here are a few examples from each list:

Things I Want in a Dating Relationship
- Reciprocity (the phone works both ways)
- Independence (alone time)
- Dependability and adult maturity

Things I Don't Want in a Dating Relationship
- Manipulation
- Neediness/dependency
- To lose myself

After I wrote these lists, I forgot about them completely. When I first met Mark, I never referred to them at all. In fact, I didn't even find them in my journal until after I had called off the wedding. Today I have updated lists hanging on my refrigerator, and I refer to them frequently. (Tools only work when you use them.)

Make similar lists of your own. If you are not dating, refer to your lists when you begin that journey. (This is a journey you must be ready for, so you might want to talk with your therapist about it.) If you already have someone special in your life, use your lists to make sure your current relationship is congruent with your values. Make necessary changes.

You Asked About My Family

MANY OF YOU have asked, "What about your family?" So here's a bit about the Schaefers, who lived for most of my childhood at 360 Oak Trail Drive in a suburb of Dallas, Texas. It was my dad; my mom; my two brothers, Steven (two years older) and Jeffery (four years younger); and me (yes, the middle child).

Let's start with my dad, Joe. My dad is smart, loving, and a great parent. (Ditto for my mom.) He worked as a chemical engineer for more than thirty years to support our family, but he was home by 5:30 P.M. to eat dinner with us. Prior to my telling him about Ed, he didn't know what an eating disorder was or what to say to someone who had one. One of the first things he did say was "Why don't you just eat three meals a day like your mother and I do?"

To an engineer, this seemed logical, like the smart thing to do. My dad is a quick learner, and he soon realized that my eating disorder was about much more than just food. He was willing to do whatever it took to help me, including paying for treatment and driving from Texas to Tennessee to participate in family therapy.

My mom, Susan, joined him on all of those rides. Historically, moms get false blame for illnesses, including autism and schizophrenia. They used to get blamed for eating disorders too. It sure didn't help me when my mom read books that said she was to blame for my disorder. She felt guilty, which made me feel guilty. My mom didn't cause my eating disorder, but she did absolutely everything she could to help me get better.

Both of my parents thought that once I got help, I would recover rather quickly. I thought that too. We were all very wrong.

I'm grateful that my mom and dad stayed by my side throughout the long recovery journey.

So did my brothers. Steven listened to me cry over the phone about Ed many times. He didn't know exactly what to say, so he mostly just listened. Sometimes, he would say, "I don't understand what you're going through, but I believe you." For instance, he could never understand how I could possibly feel fat, but he believed that I really did feel that way and learned to not get us both frustrated by trying to convince me otherwise. This was always incredibly helpful to me. In fact, my entire family was in a better position to truly support me after they stopped trying so hard to understand everything. Likewise, I was in a better position to receive their support when I quit trying to explain it all.

My younger brother, Jeffery, is friends with many of you on MySpace and Facebook. I will never forget when he told me that he had felt guilty for not knowing that I had problems with food when we were growing up. He couldn't have known, but when he found out, he did everything he could to help me (even though he was a busy college student). I have to admit that Jeffery got the short end of the stick when it came to Ed. I was moody and irritable, and Jeffery was an easy target for my anger. Luckily, he was good at separating me from Ed. He always loved me. He probably hated Ed.

I had to teach my family how to support me. Before I could do that, I had to go inside and figure it out myself. I talked about it in therapy. I was twenty-two when I first entered treatment for my eating disorder and living in a different state from everyone else in my family. As long as I was getting professional help for my disorder, I told my family they didn't have to ask me about food. I just wanted them to talk to me about life.

My family didn't do anything wrong, but sometimes they didn't know exactly what to do right. Recently, my parents said that maybe they shouldn't have praised me so much for my schoolwork in middle and high school (for making straight As and studying so much), but instead should have encouraged me to have more fun. My parents never put pressure on me to be perfect, but—like any parent—they did pat me on the back for doing well. By the time college rolled around, they could see that my high, perfectionistic standards were unhealthy, and they did, in fact, encourage me to study less and play more. I remember my dad saying, "We don't want you to bring home another 4.0. Get at least a B. Even a C would be great."

One particularly helpful thing my family did was to always take care of themselves. I was trying to learn how to take care of my body, and they were incredible examples of how to do that (excluding Jeffery's not-so-smart decision to jump off a waterfall in New Zealand). Another important thing they did was to never give up on me. No matter how sick I became, no matter how many times I relapsed, they always believed that I could recover. They always loved me.

My family never understood how food—something we all need to survive—could cause so much turmoil, confusion, and pain. The good news is they never needed to. They learned what they could, they grew, and they made changes. I did too. People often talk about how eating disorders can tear families apart, but you don't hear a lot about how recovery can bring them together. My family is closer than ever.

With the help of those four people who used to live at 360 Oak Trail Drive, I did a 360—turned my life around completely. (I guess it's a good thing we didn't live at *60* Oak Trail Drive.) Thanks, Dad, Mom, Steve, and Jeff!

My Mentee

I ALREADY FEEL A special connection with my newborn nephew, Aiden, because—just like me—he is the middle child. His parents, Steven and Destiny, might disagree with my saying that he is the middle child, since he is really only the second of two kids. A minor technicality. Naturally, I assume they will have at least one more kid for Aunt Jenni to spoil.

Recently Steven and Destiny asked me if I would be Aiden's official mentor in life. I was honored and ecstatic. I thought, "Wow! I sure have come a long way if parents are actually asking me to mentor their child."

Needless to say, when Ed and I were married, parents weren't exactly running up to me on the street asking me to guide their children. But today I'm ready to be Aiden's mentor. I will be a good one too, thanks to the various mentors I've had in my life.

When I first sought help for my eating disorder, one of my mentors was Emily, a young woman who had recovered from anorexia and bulimia. At one time, she was my sponsor in a Twelve Step program for eating disorders, and she regularly shared her experience, strength, and hope with me. If she could recover, I could too. Connecting face-to-face with Emily was crucial for my successful recovery.

During therapy, I was actually encouraged to have a make-believe mentor. Scarlett O'Hara, in the classic movie *Gone with the Wind* (1939), was someone I had looked up to since I was a teenager. I admired how she challenged the traditional gender roles in her society. She was passionate, strong, and assertive. Since I often did therapy work on being more assertive, in certain situations, it would help to ask myself, "What would Scarlett do?" By practicing this over and over, and with continued personal growth work, I ultimately learned to trust myself and ask, "What would Jenni do?"

Vivien Leigh, the actress who played Scarlett, also became a role model. She shared many of the characteristics that I admired in Scarlett. She also courageously battled bipolar disorder at a time when the illness was even more misunderstood than it is now. I personally came to understand bipolar disorder better through Marya Hornbacher's powerful book, *Madness*. And Marya is yet another mentor. One day, like her, I hope to write about a wide array of topics.

Today I have mentors in all areas of my life, such as in the publishing world, the eating disorder field, and the music business. I have spiritual mentors. My mom and dad are mentors. I speak with some of my mentors regularly, while others I have never met. Regardless of whether or not these people know they are my mentors, and regardless of whether or not they are even real people, they are all helping me to become a better person.

I hope that I can do that for Aiden too. When this book is released, Aiden still won't be anywhere close to reading. (Although I guess it's possible that I will be such a great mentor that he'll be reading books by one and a half.)

Aiden, whenever you can finally read these words, thank you. Thank you for letting me guide you. In doing so, I'm continually taking steps in the right direction for myself.

In this way, my mentee is also my mentor.

Real Action: Do You Have a Mentor?

A Recovery Mentor

Many of you have e-mailed me to say, "Jenni, I have never personally met anyone who is recovered from an eating disorder."

Just because you've never met anyone doesn't mean they aren't out there. They are! I have met countless women and men who are fully recovered. Do your best to find a role model who is recovered—someone you can witness first-hand living a happy, healthy, recovered life and someone you can connect with face-to-face.

Go to Twelve Step meetings or attend an eating disorder therapy group. Talk with your therapist about your desire to connect with someone who lives a genuinely recovered life. Remember that a recovery mentor is not a replacement for therapy, but can be an important adjunct to it.

You might want to read Shannon Cutts's book, *Beating Ana*, which specifically talks about connecting with others along the road to recovery.

Other Mentors in Your Life

Whom do you look up to? We all need people in our lives to serve as mentors, coaches, and role models. These people don't have to be perfect. It's okay to choose those whom you respect for certain attributes even if you appreciate other qualities about them less. Your mentors can be real people (living today or long ago), or they can be fictional (like Scarlett O'Hara).

Be creative. Choose mentors who can really inspire you to be the best person you can be. Sooner or later, don't be surprised when someone asks you to be a mentor yourself!

I Am a Mind Reader

I AM A MIND reader. I can predict what people are thinking and feeling. I know, pretty impressive, huh? There's only one slight problem with my skills. My predictions are almost always wrong.

I remember first coming to terms with the fact that I am a mind reader—and a bad one at that—in a family therapy session almost ten years ago. I had the opportunity to ask my parents direct questions about various topics. These were questions that I had never actually asked before but had predicted the answers to myself. I finally asked things like: "Are you mad at me for this? Do you not want me to do that? Do you want me to do this?"

Ultimately, all of my questions had a similar answer. My parents might not approve of everything I do, but they respect that I'm an adult living on my own who is capable of making her own decisions. They also said that there is nothing I could ever do to make them stop loving me. Nothing. I had never doubted that my parents loved me, but I had never fully grasped the idea that I am a unique person separate from them. Many of my false predictions had been based on the lie that I was simply an extension of them. The truth is that my parents wanted me to flourish as an individual. One hour of therapy broke through years of ineffective mind reading with my parents.

All in all, recovery from my eating disorder helped me to be a much better communicator in all types of situations. Likewise, becoming a better communicator helped me strengthen my recovery.

Mind reading often pushed me into Ed's arms. I worried about what people were thinking, and I turned to Ed to reduce my anxiety. When I stopped mind reading and practiced direct communication, I didn't need Ed to deal with this anxiety. (Of course, in the beginning, I was anxious about direct communication as well, but it became more comfortable with experience.) Years after that particular family session, I'm better at talking openly and honestly with my parents and others. I'm also recovered.

I remember my mom calling a few years ago to tell me that my dad had been diagnosed with cancer. She said that the prognosis was great and my dad should be fine. The mind reading part of me was activated and thought, "She's lying to protect you. Everything is not going to be fine." Instead of falling into the mind reading trap, I decided to ask my mom directly, "Are you telling me the truth, or are things really worse?" She said, "I'm telling you the truth." I chose to believe her, and she was right. My dad is now healthy.

Today I do my best to take things that people say and do at face value. Since I'm not perfect, I still catch myself playing mind reading games sometimes. For instance, if you don't respond to an e-mail I send to you within a certain amount of time, the mind reader will say that you're mad at me or, even worse, that you hate me. Heck, if you say "Good-bye," instead of "Talk to you later," the mind reader will tell me that you hate me and never want to speak to me again. (If you had wanted to talk with me again, you would have said, "Talk to you later.") The difference between the past and the present is that I now know how to get in touch with my heart, experience the moment, and recognize the truth. The truth is I'm not a mind reader after all.

Lonely

L IVING ALONE IS great. I don't find empty milk cartons in my refrigerator, and I can usually find the remote control. An added bonus: I never fall into the toilet! But lately, I've been thinking that, every once in a while, it might actually be nice to have someone else around, at least in the other room. Sometimes I feel lonely.

Did I just say that? It still feels weird for me to say or write the word *lonely*. (Yes, weird is good.) Prior to Ed packing his bags, *lonely* was not a part of my vocabulary. In fact, when people used to say, "I feel lonely," it was as if they were speaking a foreign language. My brain translated "I feel lonely" into "I'm weak." I equated loneliness with weakness, and I took pride in the fact that I never felt lonely.

As it turns out, guess who was actually very lonely? Me. With Ed as my constant companion, I just wasn't in touch with feeling lonely.

Ed masked those feelings while simultaneously creating an environment in which I was ultimately more and more alone. He wanted me all to himself—thriving on isolation—so he said that I needed only him and encouraged me to push other people away. I would frequently go for days at a time without any significant human interaction (for example, talking only with the bank teller or the grocery store clerk). I didn't begin to realize how isolated from the world I was until I kicked Ed out of my life for good. With him gone, I discovered loneliness—all kinds and varying degrees of it.

Sometimes I felt lonely because I had pushed people away for so long that I honestly didn't have many close connections left. I was physically isolated and disconnected from the world. Sometimes I felt lonely in a crowded room. This kind of loneliness pierced my soul and ached to the core. I not only felt disconnected from the world, but I also felt like no one loved me. Intellectually, I knew that people did, but I still felt that way.

I have made a lot of changes in my life to help deal with loneliness. First and foremost, I accept that loneliness is a natural and normal part of the human condition. I experience the feelings without stuffing myself or starving them away. I have learned strategies for nurturing myself when I feel lonely. Sometimes I take myself out on dates alone. I do what I would do with others—rent a movie or take a stroll in the park—even if no one else is around. When I feel lonely sitting at my desk writing, I pack up my laptop and head to the nearest coffee shop. Even if I don't speak with anyone, I still feel like a part of the larger coffee shop community.

I have also worked to create a network of people in my life. I have reconnected with old friends and made new ones. Interdependence, not independence, is now my goal. With old and new friends, I now initiate social events instead of always waiting for others to call me. Sometimes I even anticipate times when I might feel lonely (like during the holidays) and schedule something to look forward to with others. When I experience deep feelings of loneliness for long periods of time, I talk it over with Ann and seek medical help if necessary.

So here I am, writing this section while sitting alone in my home. I am alone today, but I don't feel lonely. Loneliness is different from solitude. I treasure moments of solitude like this that energize me. But when I do feel lonely, I recognize that it is actually progress. Unlike what I used to believe, feeling lonely is not a sign of weakness, but of strength. It means that I'm connecting with my feelings and accepting the present moment. When you feel lonely, know that I understand. In our loneliness, strangely, we are connected.

Hang-Up Syndrome

IF YOU KNEW me while I was working on being more assertive, you were probably the recipient of a hang-up. This means that during one of our phone conversations, I probably angrily slammed the phone down while you were in midsentence because I didn't like what you were saying and I was trying to be assertive. I hung up on you. You weren't very happy about that.

I understand why. Hanging up on people is disrespectful; it is not assertive. As I transitioned from being everyone's doormat to being a confident person able to express my own opinions, I definitely swung the pendulum a little too far past assertive to that place called rude. Finding the middle ground took practice and time. Thank you for being patient with me.

My treatment team told me that my new diagnosis of hang-up syndrome was actually progress for me. It meant that I was attempting to express my true self and desires as opposed to my old pattern of using Ed to communicate, stuffing my feelings, and simply saying things to please others. It went something like this: Ed would say, "You're angry with Sally, so you better restrict today. That will show her!" So I would starve myself, all the while telling Sally (with a smile) something I thought she wanted to hear. Then I would resent Sally, and Ed would encourage me to binge to deal with the resentment. It seemed like a never-ending cycle.

I got tired of banging my head against the same wall. (The wall wouldn't break, and my head got really sore.) I began to realize that to experience true independence from Ed, I was going to have to start using my voice—not bingeing, purging, and restricting— to communicate. I was going to have to start expressing my needs in a clear and confident manner. Speaking my truth meant stretching past my comfort zone. In the beginning, it also meant that instead of being clear and confident, I was sometimes rude and confusing.

I would get so frustrated trying to express myself that—out of nowhere—I would just slam the phone down (loudly). With continued practice in being assertive and not aggressive, and getting feedback in individual and group therapy, these surprise-attack hang-ups eventually became planned hang-ups. Instead of cutting someone off in midsentence, I would politely say, "I'm so mad that I'm going to hang up on you now." And *then* I would disconnect.

Progress, yes. But I obviously needed to go further. I kept practicing being assertive with my treatment team and with the women in my therapy group. These were people I could trust to give me room to grow. I practiced being more assertive with my family, whom I could also trust.

All of this practice falling down and getting back up again brought me to where I am today. I no longer resemble a doormat for other people; I stand up for myself. I don't always do this perfectly, but for the most part, I can state my needs clearly and effectively without being aggressive or passive. I now understand that people can't read my mind, just like I can't read theirs.

People in my life have had to get used to the new me. Ironically, many of the people who originally encouraged me to be more assertive actually didn't like the new, confident me. Over time, many of them grew to accept and even love my new and improved version, while others slipped out of my life.

I now surround myself with self-confident people who like to be around others with confidence. Find the self-assurance that lives within you and join us. Just give me a call. I won't hang up on you. Promise.

Personal Protected Days

PRIOR TO GOING out last night, I received a text from Amy, a friend who is in recovery from an eating disorder. The message read, "I can't go out tonight with you after all. I need to practice self-care and take a night to relax. My doctor calls it 'couch time.'"

I remembered back to when I was first learning how to take alone time for myself, and I completely understood why she had chosen her couch over me.

When I was in early recovery, instead of couch time, I talked about personal protected days, or PPDs for short. These were specified days each week (I usually chose Tuesday and Thursday) when I would carve out a few hours for myself—hence the first *P* in PPD stands for *personal*.

My goal in therapy was to have two PPDs per week. Since I worked during the daytime Monday through Friday, I usually set aside time for myself in the evening. (In this way, I suppose that my personal protected days were actually nights.) On those nights I relaxed, rejuvenated, and connected with myself. If I wanted to read a book and light candles, I did that. If I wanted to write, I did that. The key to a good PPD was doing whatever I wanted, not necessarily what I needed to do. If what I wanted was also something that I needed to do, like washing dishes, I did it. I'm one of those people who actually like to unload the dishwasher. I do not like to vacuum, so my floors were never particularly clean on personal protected days.

The second *P* in PPD stands for *protected*, because I had to work hard to protect these nights. There was always someone who tried to impinge on this personal space, even if they had the best of intentions. I had to practice saying no and risk disappointing others to protect my personal time. This may sound strange, but I also had to protect this time from myself. There was always something I should have been doing instead of what I wanted to do. I *should* have been going to the office party, helping a friend, or whatever else, and I often felt I was being selfish if I chose alone time over these things. I learned that taking time for myself is not selfish, but necessary. The key to PPDs was connecting with what I really wanted, protecting that time, and sometimes literally forcing myself to do it.

As someone who is prone to isolation, I also had to make sure that I was using PPDs in a healthy way, the way my treatment team and I had discussed. I couldn't use them as an excuse to avoid making friends or to miss out on group or individual therapy. I had to use them as a tool to balance my life. Personal protected days taught me how to keep a healthy amount of alone time in my new life while also trying to connect more genuinely with others. What I have learned about myself is that if I don't get enough alone time, then I don't appreciate and enjoy the time I have with others. Instead, I become resentful and am not a lot of fun to be around. PPDs were all about incorporating balance into my life.

Today I still need private time to be at my healthiest, happiest, and most productive. I don't use the term PPD anymore, because carving out time for myself has become more intuitive (something I do naturally) after years of practice. There are certainly periods when I don't get enough alone time, and I feel it quickly—both physically and emotionally. During these times, I look at my schedule, work hard and fast to create some me time, and try to prioritize it the same way that I would a dentist appointment (which I always set six months in advance and stick with). I try not to create me time out of time that is left over or that I can find between other tasks. I set aside real quality time so I can genuinely feel a benefit.

We all need different amounts of alone time based on our personalities, schedules, and family commitments. Even if you live with a friend, a spouse, a partner, or kids, it is important to find some space for yourself. My friend Sandi is a single mother, and she has taught her young children to respect her alone time, which they call "mommy time."

No matter what you call it—couch time, PPD, me time, alone time, mommy time, or something else—make sure that you get it. Do whatever it takes to find this space and protect it.

If it means canceling plans with me, I will understand.

Real Action: Protect Time with Yourself

Look at your calendar and schedule a PPD for yourself. Set aside some quality time for yourself. This might be a weeknight after work or school, or possibly an afternoon over the weekend. Do something you have wanted to do for a while but never had the time. Now you *do* have the time!

Here's the really hard part: do it again and again. Make PPDs a part of your life.

Making Friends

SARAH DIDN'T HAVE many friends because she had been through a divorce in which her husband "took" the friends and she got the house. Danny didn't have close friends because he had put his energy into romantic relationships rather than friendships. Cindy didn't have good friends because Ed had been her one and only friend for so long.

Does any of this sound familiar? It did to me, and not that long ago. People thought I had lots of close friends, because I had a popular book out and I was on the television and radio a lot. Let me tell you what was really going on.

During recovery, the only friends I saw on a regular basis were the girls in my therapy group. As we became healthier, the goal was to not have perfect attendance in group. We drifted apart, and I headed straight into an engagement with Mark and spent most of my time with him. After we broke up, I found myself incredibly isolated. I knew I needed to make real, meaningful connections with people, but how?

I first focused on people who were already in my life. I began letting friends in on a whole new level, letting them get to know the real me. I began to let people help me, and I reached out to help others as well. I made a conscious effort to spend quality time with friends. I had often used my travel schedule as an excuse for not hanging out with others, saying, "I'm only in town two days next week, so I can't get together." I began to say, "I'm only in town two days next week, so let's get together then."

I began to notice that most of my friends empowered me. They made me feel good inside. I was a better person because of them. These friendships were reciprocal without anyone having to keep score (that "I did this for you, so you owe me" mentality). These friendships were based on direct communication and love, not codependency. (These were *not* the people who removed me as a Top Friend on MySpace to tell me they were upset with me.)

A handful of people in my life were more like energy vampires. They didn't lift me up; they pulled me down. I had to "break up" with these people and focus on spending more time with those who empowered me.

Making true friends is kind of like dating in that it doesn't always work out with someone, and that's okay. Holding myself to perfectionistic standards, I used to think I had to become lifelong friends with everyone who entered my life. This was exhausting, and I now know it's not true. I believe the old saying that people come into your life for a reason, a season, or a lifetime.

I have talked with many people in recovery who say they have had to distance themselves for periods of time from certain friends who are struggling with eating disorders, because their Eds were becoming closer than they were. (Rather than building the friendship, each person's eating disorder was getting bigger.)

In addition to strengthening the positive relationships I already had (and ending the negative ones), I made new friends. One day I was talking with my friend Rob about my difficulty in this area. He pointed out that I first needed to be open to it. He knew I was going to a social event that night where I might meet people, so he gave me an assignment. He asked me to introduce myself to three people and to e-mail him their first names and something about each of them in the morning. I agreed and quickly uncovered some of my difficulties in meeting people.

One negative pattern was that I would go to social events late, leave early, and not make much of an effort to talk with anyone while I was there. (You don't meet many people this way.) I also discovered that I appeared physically closed off, standing with my arms crossed and avoiding eye contact. I have had to concentrate on changing my body language, looking into people's eyes, and smiling. It was difficult that night, but I did meet three people.

Rob's assignment reminded me that I generally need to be more open to introducing myself to others, finding out their names, and asking them about themselves.

Something I have learned from talking to people with eating disorders is that many of us feel socially awkward when we first start hanging out in the "real world." Sometimes we think everyone is analyzing our weight and watching what we eat. (I discovered that most people are too absorbed in their own lives to actually notice changes in my weight or pay attention to what I have for dinner.) Sometimes we don't know what to say in conversations because we have been talking with and about Ed for so long. In the beginning, I actually had to concentrate on not talking about Ed so much and on discussing other things in my life. I eventually learned to just be myself.

I am surrounded by wonderful people today. I'm also a better friend. I have learned that listening is an active, not a passive, process. Hearing people is different from listening to them. I have discovered what it means to be trustworthy. Keeping secrets means keeping secrets. It doesn't mean passing one along and saying, "I'm not supposed to tell you this, so don't tell anyone, but . . ." Being a good friend means being honest. I have learned this too.

If your heart aches for real relationships, you will probably discover what I did: there are many people out there who want to make friends just as much as you do. These people will be lucky to call you friend.

If you run into me somewhere, please introduce yourself! I will do the same.

5

THE WHITE DRESS

A Healthy Body and Positive Body Image

I did not have to walk down the aisle in a white dress for my inner marriage of mind, body, and spirit. But I did have to learn how to walk through my life in a new body. Regardless of my size and shape, my age, society's opinion, or anything else, I had to develop a healthy attitude and healthy feelings toward my body. I had to learn how to nourish it properly with food and exercise. Today I can honestly say that I love my body. Part 5 will help you love and cherish your body too—just the way it is.

The Worst Pickup Line Ever

I RECENTLY HEARD THE worst pickup line I can imagine. A guy approached me in the gym the other day, looked me up and down, and said, "It looks like you're here to lose weight too."

Yes, he really did say that! I actually laughed and said, "No, I'm not here to lose anything. I'm here to gain muscle and bone." I was lifting weights as prescribed by my doctor to combat osteoporosis, which is a weakening of the bones I had developed as a result of my eating disorder.

Since I didn't jump right into one of those all-too-common-in-our-society body-loathing conversations, the guy felt rejected, turned around, and walked away. As he left, I wondered why he hadn't just said hi and asked for my phone number. I let his comment just roll off my back.

But after I left the gym and returned home, I found myself wondering if he truly thought I needed to lose weight. Did he think my legs were too big? Or was it my arms? I looked at my body in the bathroom mirror and heard a voice inside my head say, "You could stand to lose a few pounds." I quickly recognized these negative thoughts and said, "Back off, Ed!"

Or *was* it Ed? Talking to him like this no longer felt congruent with my personal experience of being fully recovered. I didn't struggle with an eating disorder anymore, so why was I still talking to Ed? Why was I still giving him a place in my life?

I explained the entire situation to Ann, who has never had an eating disorder. She said that hearing a comment like that from a guy in the gym would have made her feel the same way I had. She would have started scrutinizing her body immediately—even before leaving the gym—and heard the same voice saying, "You could stand to lose a few pounds."

I thought to myself, "If Ann has never had an eating disorder and she hears the same voice in her head that I do, then the voice I sometimes hear today must not be Ed."

I looked at Ann with a confused expression and said, "I'm fully recovered from my eating disorder, so the Ed idea doesn't seem to work for me anymore." Referring to the situation in the gym, I continued, "It didn't feel right for me to talk with Ed that day, because my eating disorder wasn't really talking to me. I was just experiencing some momentary negative feelings about my body, like almost anyone would have after being asked by a total stranger if she were trying to lose weight."

Ann understood and replied, "Instead of calling that voice Ed, maybe you should rename it to make it true for you now. What do you want to call that voice?"

Just because I once had an eating disorder, it doesn't mean I have to call that voice Ed forever. I have a new reality now. After thinking about Ann's question for a few months, I finally came up with an answer that fits my new life.

Strangely, the worst pickup line ever has helped me formulate the best vision of my recovered life. I decided to call that voice that we all hear in today's image-obsessed world Societal Ed.

Societal Ed

"I DON'T HAVE AN eating disorder, but I have an Ed," said Kelly.

Stuart said the same thing. So did Bob, Nicole, Chandra, and many others. After reading *Life Without Ed*, lots of people who have never had an eating disorder, who have healthy relationships with food and their bodies, tell me that "an Ed" lives in their heads. As I noted in the last section, I call this voice Societal Ed.

Societal Ed tells us—regardless of whether or not we have ever had an eating disorder—that our bodies aren't good enough and that we need to look more like the unrealistic images that appear in movies, magazines, and television series. To get this unattainable body, he tells us to do whatever we have to do—namely, overexercise and undereat. He tells us to divide food into good and bad categories and to eat only those in the good category. Of course, this category changes depending on the latest fad diet. This voice is one reason the dieting industry is so financially successful despite its actual lack of success in helping people lose weight.

Societal Ed talks loudly to men and woman, adults and children. His voice is especially strong in the United States and other Western cultures (where everything from billboards to radio ads reinforces it), and no one seems to be immune from seeing and hearing his message. Only extreme isolation (like living underground or in a cave somewhere) could prevent exposure. We all hear Societal Ed, but we don't all have to listen.

I listened to him when I was only four years old. Looking back, I can see that he helped open the door for my personal Ed to start running the show. But thanks to my work in recovery, I don't listen anymore. In fact, because I spent so many years in therapy working on developing healthy eating habits and a positive body image, I know many more ways to deal with Societal Ed than most of my "normal" friends who have never struggled with an eating disorder. They've never had the opportunity to talk with trained professionals for hours each week about the size of their hips or attend a therapy group to learn how to eat a hamburger without guilt. Because I have, I can see through Societal Ed's lies and don't let him affect me.

Sure, sometimes when I look in the bathroom mirror, he wants me to believe that my body isn't good enough, so he might say something like, "You could stand to lose a little weight."

In these moments, my friend and colleague, Anita Johnston, Ph.D., author of *Eating in the Light of the Moon*, taught me to look in the mirror with curiosity rather than fear. So I may look at my reflection and think, "That's interesting. I wonder why my body seems bigger today than it did yesterday. Maybe it's water weight. Maybe it's my outfit. Or maybe my eyes are just playing tricks on me."

I know it's not possible for me to gain a noticeable amount of weight overnight, so I will go no further than that. I move on with my day without skipping a beat—and definitely without missing a meal.

Instead of being afraid and focusing on the outside, I will ulti-mately go inside and think, "What am I feeling right now? What do I need right now?" I know the answers to these questions do not involve weight, and I connect with my heart.

When I hear Societal Ed speak to me these days, sometimes it means that something completely unrelated to my body and weight is going on in my life and I need to take a closer look at that. So I pay extra attention to my feelings and to getting my needs met.

Thanks to all of my work in recovery from my own personal Ed, Societal Ed doesn't have the power to control my actions or even my moods. When I confront him today, it reminds me of how grateful I am to be recovered from an eating disorder.

It is important to note that I didn't make the distinction between Societal Ed and my personal Ed until after I had fully recovered. I'm able to make the distinction now because talking about Ed in relation to normal body image issues no longer feels right to me. Just because I had an eating disorder at one time doesn't mean that the normal body image stuff I (and almost everyone else) experience today is anorexia and bulimia. I refuse to keep defining myself in those terms. I will not give Ed a place in my life. Our culture continues to give Societal Ed a place in our world, but I choose not to let him live in my mind either. What will you choose?

What if I Never Stop Eating?

"WHAT IF INTUITIVE eating doesn't work for me? What if I start eating again and never stop gaining weight? What if I never stop eating?" These were questions I had about this thing called intuitive eating. Needless to say, the transition process from my food plan to intuitive eating was not a piece of cake. (I did learn how to eat cake though.)

Getting in touch with my hunger and fullness cues was quite a challenge. When Ed was running the show, I thought hunger was that place I sometimes reached when my stomach actually ached and growled. I thought fullness was when my stomach hurt from being stuffed with binge food. No body should have to reach these extremes.

In recovery, I learned subtle ways to tell if I'm hungry or full. I might be hungry if I find myself craving a particular food, and I might be getting full if a certain food no longer tastes as good. I learned that it's normal to feel pressure in my body when I'm full. It's normal for my pants to fit differently. This does not mean I'm fat, but that I'm full. There is a difference.

After I became more in touch with these cues, trusting my body was a major hurdle. If I felt hungry, I knew my body needed food. But could I really trust it with food? If I gave myself permission to eat, Ed told me that anything might happen. I might never stop eating.

During the worst stages of my eating disorder, I was all-or-none with food—either bingeing or not eating. Much of my experience was, in fact, that if I ate anything, I would eat everything. I began to understand that this happened because I was starving myself. In starvation mode, my body literally thought I was facing a famine. It didn't know that I was living near a grocery store and several fast-food restaurants. Thinking I was facing a real food shortage, its primal instinct was to binge on large amounts of food, conserving fat in preparation for the hard times ahead. I began to understand this concept better when I learned about the starvation study performed by Ancel Keys, Ph.D.

During World War II, Dr. Keys researched the human body's reaction to starvation to determine how best to refeed millions of starving war victims. From a group of American conscientious objectors to the war, he recruited young male volunteers who were in their prime both physically and psychologically. When starved, these once-healthy men displayed symptoms similar to those associated with anorexia and bulimia. Metabolic rates dropped, while food obsessions skyrocketed. The men reported binge eating, depression, decreased concentration, fatigue, irritability, feeling cold, and more. I experienced the same things with Ed. (A particularly wonderful gift of recovery is that I'm no longer cold all the time.)

During the refeeding period of the experiment when the men could eat freely again, many reported that their hunger was insatiable. They couldn't stop eating. Some said that the refeeding period was even more difficult than the starvation period. It took the majority of men months for their eating habits to average out. And they hadn't been anxious about gaining weight because Ed was yelling in their ear all along the way, as people struggling with eating disorders are. Dr. Keys's study taught me that I needed to be patient with myself. My body had reacted normally to being starved, and I would have to give it time to become healthy again. It would be difficult, but I could do it.

Another challenge I experienced with intuitive eating was my tendency to undereat, which always set me up to binge. When I finally committed to adding more food to the mix, I erred on the side of overdoing it for a while. I think I was so excited that food was legal that I just wanted to eat more and more. And for a time, I ate mostly foods that had once been forbidden. This scared me for a while, but I stayed the course, and the overeating eventually evened out to intuitive eating. An important point is that I don't think undereating would ever have evened out; it would have just kept me stuck. As my eating became balanced, my weight did too.

Ever since I can remember, I thought I was born to be fat. To maintain the weight I wanted, I believed I would always have to restrict. I was wrong. Intuitive eating has given me the body I truly want. You won't see me walking down the runway as a model, but you might see me climbing frozen waterfalls in Alaska. That's where I'd rather be anyway.

To answer the question, "What if I never stop eating?" I never intend on stopping. I intend to eat every day for the rest of my life in an intuitive way. Today eating every day is not a nightmare. It's freedom.

No, I will never stop eating, not again.

Supercute

A COUPLE DAYS AGO, I went to a singles event called Solo on the Patio. Since I didn't really want to be solo on the patio, I went with a couple of girlfriends. When we arrived—as a trio—we looked supercute.

After male solos rejected me (and not necessarily either of my younger girlfriends) all night long, I didn't feel so supercute. I felt superfat, superold, and superugly. The difference between today and years ago is that feeling superbad didn't make me want to supersize anything. I didn't want to binge. Turning to food didn't even cross my mind. Instead, I turned inside.

I asked myself, "Why do I feel fat, old, and ugly?"

Let's start with feeling fat. Thanks to years of attending individual therapy, eating disorder group therapy, and even a body image group, I have honed my skills in handling that fat feeling that creeps into most people's lives from time to time—whether or not they have ever had an eating disorder. (As I pointed out earlier, Societal Ed likes to tell us that we are not the right size or shape.)

I've heard it said that fat is not really a feeling. Well, it sure feels like a feeling, because it covers up real feelings. These days, when I feel fat, I ask myself, "What am I feeling beneath that?"

The night of Solo on the Patio, I discovered that I was feeling lonely and sad. So before going to sleep, I was gentle with myself. I called a friend, took a relaxing bath, and curled up in bed with a good book. When I woke up, the fat feeling was gone.

But the old and ugly feelings were still there. Luckily, I realized that I had a therapy appointment already scheduled for that morning. (Don't you love it when that happens?) I explained everything to Ann and discovered that feeling old and feeling ugly were linked for me.

Amid a bunch of twenty-somethings at the singles event, I felt old. I noticed that men of all ages seemed to approach only the very young women. As a thirty-two-year-old, I'm in this strange land where I am sometimes labeled young and sometimes old. That night, I was labeled old. (Pay particular attention to the word *labeled*.) Some men labeled me as old, and I took it on. By accepting that label, I also accepted the common view of what it means for a woman to be old and felt ugly. In our society, we are taught incorrectly that men get more distinguished with age and women just get ugly.

I was surprised at my experience with feeling old that night, because I had just spent a good part of the day (prior to the patio event) giving my friend Melanie, who had just turned thirty, a pep talk about getting older. She was really down about hitting the big three-oh, so I told her that I'm happier and healthier than ever in my thirties. I also said that age has brought me wisdom, insight, and clarity that can only be gained from life experience, not from some textbook.

I explained that age is the common denominator. We all get one day older every day—no exceptions. Why fight something you can't change? Why not celebrate it instead? I told Melanie that I refuse to get older. I would never want to go back to my younger years. Never!

Only a few hours later, at the singles event, I found myself wishing I were younger. I was surprised that a small part of me is still so attached to society's view of aging. Ann encouraged me to connect with my heart and think about what I want my life to stand for. I thought about one of Maya Angelou's lines: "Don't just be an aging female—become a real woman."

I want to be a real woman. The reality is that some men are attracted to younger women (especially men at a singles event on a Tuesday night). The reality is that Western society applauds youth and looks down on age. <u>My reality is that I'm as young as I feel. Youth is a perspective.</u> Age is a point of view. <u>Supercute is a state of mind.</u>

Regardless of your specific age, or whether you're a man or woman, make a decision to embrace the truth and empower yourself. Rather than adding to society's distorted views, we can all support each other in being real.

Each year, with the help of those around me, I am learning how to be a better, stronger woman—a real woman. And a supercute one at that!

Real Action: What Do You Want Your Life to Stand For?

When I was worried about society's view of aging, Ann asked me what I wanted my life to stand for. Take some time to answer this question for yourself.

Sunny Day Versus Dark Knight

I WAS ALL DRESSED to go hiking in Nashville to enjoy a sunny day. I was walking out the door, headed to my favorite park, when my friend Georgia called to see if I wanted to go with her and Dave to see *The Dark Knight*. I didn't have time to go hiking and see the movie, so the question became "sunny day or *Dark Knight*?"

Without much hesitation, I said, "Sure," changed my clothes, and headed to the movie theater. On another day, I might have chosen to go outside instead.

These days, I intuitively know what I want to do when it comes to things like this. On that sunny day, I needed to be with friends more than I needed to go hiking. So *The Dark Knight* it was. Years ago, of course, Ed would have insisted that I choose hiking over sitting still in a movie theater.

This may surprise you, but there is such a thing as intuitive exercise. It involves listening to your body and knowing what it needs in regard to physical activity. If I slow down enough and listen inwardly, I can actually detect what my body wants. I can tell whether I want to go hiking, biking, or walking—or lie on the couch and do nothing.

I actually began struggling with compulsive exercise after I entered recovery, not before. I went through a phase in which I thought I had to exercise every single day, no matter what. This is not the case. In fact, there is such a thing as too much exercise, which can actually hurt your body.

Since Ed wasn't going to confess back then, I had to talk honestly with my treatment team about my exercise patterns. Slowly, over time, they guided me toward intuitive exercise. In the process, I asked myself questions like, "Why do I want to go to the gym today?" My motive became more about health, well-being, and fun rather than calorie burning. I had to make sure I was eating enough to accommodate any physical activity. If I was injured or sick, I had to take time off from exercise completely. Even if I wasn't injured or sick, I still needed to be able to take time off, to turn down exercise for a movie with friends.

The Dark Knight was an incredible movie, and the popcorn was especially good that day. Ed sure would have hated that combination: sedentary activity plus popcorn. But he doesn't have to like it. I did! So did Georgia and Dave.

A Thigh of Relief

M Y THIGHS TOUCH. When I stand up straight with my feet together, my thighs touch at the top. I used to hate not having any space between my thighs, but not anymore. Today I love it. I'm serious. Read on.

When I was lost in my eating disorder, I would stand in front of my bathroom mirror each morning and night to make sure my thighs didn't touch. (I now understand that this is not the most productive way to spend my time.) Since I was at an unnaturally thin weight, they never came into contact, and I would let out a big sigh of relief.

After getting professional help, I gained some much-needed weight, but I was still too thin for my body type. (I struggled for years to maintain an unnaturally low weight while simultaneously trying to be recovered. This doesn't work.) With the added weight, it took lots of strategic effort, but I could still position my legs in such a way that my thighs wouldn't meet. I would let out an even bigger sigh of relief. For me, this was a tool by which I falsely measured happiness, success, and self-worth.

Today no amount of strategizing prevents my thighs from touching. I'm at my body's "set point weight," which is more of a range than a specific number. I think of my set point as my ideal weight, my natural weight, and my healthy weight. It's where my body genetically wants to be and where it fights to be despite any efforts to go lower or higher. When I weighed lower than my set point, my body fought back by slowing my metabolism and giving me intense cravings to binge on large amounts of food—both attempts to increase my weight.

Because I tried to control my weight for so long in destructive ways, it took a long time (even after I began eating well) for my weight to even out and get to where it is now. In the process, I actually weighed more than my set point for a short time. Finally, at my natural weight, my metabolism is normal, I am in touch with my hunger and fullness cues, and I don't get the urge to binge. I feel energetic, healthy, and happy!

I no longer try to achieve an unrealistically thin ideal for my body type. With my proportions, including the width of my hips, I cannot possibly have space between my thighs and be at a healthy weight—and I no longer care. Other people's bodies might be made differently. I have a friend whose legs are naturally spaced farther apart than mine, and her thighs have never touched, even at a healthy weight. Magazines tell us that we should all look the same even though we're not all made the same.

You might not believe this, but I would rather be at my set point weight than anything lower. Even if a genie popped out of a bottle and could make me weigh less and still be recovered (it would take that kind of magic), I would choose to weigh what I do today. I actually think my body looks best at this weight. I have curves! I like feeling like a woman. I like feeling strong and power-ful. And I like being a good role model to others. I can't very well talk about positive body image if I'm maintaining an unhealthy weight myself.

I will admit that I wasn't always so gung ho about being this weight. In fact, I was once so distraught about it that I wrecked my car in a parking garage. (My gynecologist had accidentally told me my weight at an appointment, and I lost it.) I had to look at my thighs touching for more than a year before I could even accept it, much less like it, and much, much less love it. There was no magic pill, book, or therapeutic exercise that convinced me to love my body. A lot of things were helpful, but what helped most was just patience and giving myself time to adjust to my new body. I filled my life with other things that ultimately pushed out the negative body image thoughts slowly over time. I finally have a positive body image, and it gets better all the time.

For a long time, I tried to improve my body image *before* I would eat right and maintain a healthy weight. The hard truth is that you have to eat right and maintain a healthy weight before your body image can truly improve. This means there is a period when you are in your healthy body and feel horrible. But if you just stick with it—without manipulating your food or weight—the horrible feeling subsides, and you actually begin to love your new body. If you don't stick with it, Ed will inevitably take control and drag you down again. I discovered that I couldn't do a lot to speed up positive body image, but I could sure do a lot to slow it down. (For example, obsessing about the space between my thighs slowed it down. Restricting slowed it down. Trying to fit into clothes that were too small for me—you guessed it—slowed it down.)

Do you appreciate your body at a healthy weight or only at an unnatural size? Regardless of what number you see on the scale right now (whether you need to gain weight or not), my hope is that you will make your goal to maintain your natural weight and experience the freedom that comes with it.

When I look at my happy, healthy, touching thighs, I smile. And—you guessed it—I let out the biggest sigh of relief of them all.

Real Action: Body Checking

Do you obsessively look at yourself in the mirror? Do you check the space between your thighs? Do you pinch parts of your body looking for fat? Make a list of the ways you check your body. Discuss your list with your therapist. Talk about how body checking keeps you tied to Ed. Awareness is the first step to breaking free.

Are You a Prisoner?

I WAS SENTENCED TO life in prison. I didn't wear an orange jumpsuit, but I would have liked one. I was in bad body image prison, and I only wore clothes that would hide my body and its newfound curves. After gaining much-needed weight in recovery, I had sentenced myself to life in baggy clothing. I never wore anything that actually fit me, much less shorts or swimsuits. I believed that if people knew how my body really looked, they wouldn't like me. They would look down on me for letting myself go. So I hid.

Stuck in bad body image prison, which is a term I learned from my friend and colleague, Margo Maine, Ph.D., I missed out on a lot of fun. I didn't go to pool parties, because I wouldn't dare put on a swimsuit. No volleyball, because that required shorts. I skipped lots of social events, because I didn't feel comfortable in dressy clothes. So I just stayed home in my big T-shirts and sweatpants. During this time, my mom encouraged me to wear clothes that fit. My friends did too. They asked, "Are you ever going to wear jeans again?"

"No," I thought. "I can survive without ever wearing jeans."

I could survive in bad body image prison, but I couldn't truly *live* there. I ultimately realized that I wanted to live.

Gradually I began wearing clothes that fit—like jeans, pants with belts, and shirts that didn't fall under the "big T-shirt" or "big sweatshirt" categories. People in my life immediately told me how wonderful I looked in my new clothes. I'd thought they wouldn't like me, but they were complimenting me. They were proud of me. With patience and lots of time, wearing clothes that fit well felt good and comfortable. I gave away my baggy clothes so I could embrace my new body—just as I had thrown out my "skinny" clothes years earlier when I was first trying to gain weight. (I never knew how much clothes shopping I would have to do in recovery!)

I was finally embracing my body in jeans, but I was nowhere close to embracing it in shorts or swimsuits—until I took a summer trip to Alaska where I wanted to learn how to rock climb. My friend, who was also my climbing instructor, said that I needed to wear shorts. I really wanted to rock climb, so I decided to risk it.

As I was climbing up the big rock, my friend was helping me from below. In the beginning, I was worried that he had a perfect view of my not-so-perfect legs. Then as I climbed higher and higher up the rock, I started caring more about my life (aka not falling off and crashing to the ground below) than about what my friend might or might not be thinking about my legs. When I finally reached the top, I felt a deep appreciation for the strength in those legs.

This was, in fact, a key to my overcoming negative body image: learning to appreciate what my body does for me rather than focusing on what it looks like. As a woman, my body can not only propel me up big rocks in Alaska, but it can also create life. Amazing stuff!

Months after my Alaskan trip, I went to the beach and wore shorts for almost an entire week. I also wore a swimsuit. Similar to wearing shorts, I was very self-conscious at first. I thought everyone was staring at me and laughing at my figure. Then I began to realize that most people weren't looking at me; they were snorkeling and playing in the sand. That seemed like much more fun than body loathing, so I gave it a try too.

Bad body image prison was not just about changing my wardrobe. At one point, I hated my body so much that I could barely bathe. I had to close my eyes in the shower to avoid seeing any part of myself. I went through another period in prison where I avoided mirrors at all cost. When I entered any bathroom, I would close my eyes immediately to keep from seeing my reflection. (My eyes were closed a lot.) Bad body image prison also prevented me from dating. I didn't want a man to be close enough to see or touch my body.

I'm finally out of prison, and my eyes are wide open. It turns out that I held the key to getting out the entire time. Turning the key took lots of patience and time. It took support from others and a determination to participate more freely in life's activities. As I became more involved with living, my feelings about my body changed for the better. I began to see it as a vehicle for life experiences rather than a prison.

Today I love my body and its imperfections. I feel confident. Confidence equals beauty in my book. (And this *is* my book.) I'm beautiful, and whether you realize it yet or not, you are too.

Mixed Messages and the Machine

I WAS LYING ON a flat, hard table with a big machine scanning my body from above when the technician who was working the machine (whom I will call Nancy) said, "I just started a new diet. I think it might help you too."

Why was she giving me the latest diet advice during the middle of a routine bone density scan? Between Nancy and the guy at the gym (see "The Worst Pickup Line Ever" earlier in this section), I'm starting to wonder why complete strangers begin conversations with me by talking about weight and dieting. Whatever happened to a simple "Hello. How are you doing?"

As she spoke, I realized that she knew about my history of osteoporosis and seemed to think that her fad diet could help strengthen my not-so-strong bones. What she didn't know was that my history of anorexia and bulimia was what had caused the weakened bones in the first place. As she described the evils of fast food, I thought about how many appointments with my treatment team it had taken for me to be able to walk into a fast-food restaurant and order a cheeseburger. Eating that cheeseburger was a breakthrough, something to be celebrated, not to beat myself up over.

Nancy was beating herself up. She hung her head in shame and said things like, "I used to eat [insert a "bad" food here] and [insert another "bad" food here] every week," followed by, "I was so bad."

It became clear to me that her new diet, not any specific food, was causing her to feel bad. I think she must have wanted me to feel bad too, because she pulled out a copy of her diet plan—three typed pages—and handed it over. I was surprised that a trained professional (though *not* trained in nutrition) working in a reputable hospital would pass out diet advice to me without first consulting my doctor.

Even though I let what she said go in one ear and out the other (and tossed the information in the trash as soon as I walked out the door), I knew that years ago, her words could have been damaging to my recovery—possibly even sending me into a dangerous relapse. Knowing this, I decided to share my story with her, so that she might gain a new perspective and hopefully think twice before giving unwanted and possibly harmful information to future patients.

As Nancy went on and on about restricting food, I interrupted, "I actually know all about restricting food. I'm recovered from an eating disorder." Then I described how food does not have a moral value like good or bad.

Looking somewhat relieved, Nancy said uncertainly, "Then it's okay that I ate that piece of cake over the weekend at my daughter's birthday party." Yes!

The conversation quickly turned from talk about extreme dieting to intuitive eating. Although many resources, from websites to health care professionals, encourage me to take extreme measures with food to offset certain physical conditions, I know that balance is the key for me. For instance, I have high cholesterol, which runs in my family, and some professionals consistently tell me to go on a diet. I don't think so!

I have learned to sort through the mixed messages I receive about food and weight. Now I can laugh when I look at the cover of a women's magazine and inevitably see a headline about how to lose weight next to one touting a recipe for chocolate cake. We are told, "Eat! Eat! Eat! But don't *look* like you eat."

When I hear time and again that I need to reduce the amount of fat in my diet, I remember my dietitian tirelessly working to get me to add fat to it. And I can see the truth behind a technician who tells me that I need to restrict food in order to recover from something that was caused by restricting food in the first place.

The truth is we are all caught up in an unhealthy culture where even health care professionals sometimes reflect misguided information from the dieting industry. One accurate piece of information that Nancy gave me is that my osteoporosis is getting better.

Today I do my best to listen carefully to my body, and I regularly consult with professionals whom I trust. I do what's best for my current health while taking note of my entire medical history, which includes the fact that I once struggled with a severe, life-threatening eating disorder. This doesn't take away from the fact that I'm now fully recovered. But just as it's important to know whether or not I've ever had chicken pox, recognizing that I once had an eating disorder is significant knowledge for both my doctors and me. Based on this information, my current doctor has suggested that I treat my high cholesterol in a way that does not entail drastically changing my diet. I agree.

What works for me might not work for you and vice versa. If we would just listen to our bodies instead of all those mixed messages, we wouldn't get so mixed up. So let's start listening.

Important note: Listening to Ed is *not* the same as listening to your body. If you need help separating from Ed, keep talking with your treatment team.

Thigh Cream

THIGH CREAM: To buy, or not to buy; that is the question.

I had never thought about buying thigh cream before. In fact, I didn't even know it existed until I went to one of those makeup parties (where they try to sell you products) at my friend's house recently. I was only going to support my friend in her new business venture, not to buy anything.

When the party organizer realized that I was over thirty, she pulled out various products: something for wrinkles, something else for wrinkles, and thigh cream. She showed me a flier with before-and-after pictures of a woman who had used the cream to "control unsightly cellulite." The photos were quite convincing and got me asking myself whether or not my cellulite was unsightly too. I wondered for the first time in my life if I needed to buy thigh cream to "control" it.

The fact that the thigh cream existed and was offered to me seemed to carry with it the false implication that I needed help. I'm not easily swayed into buying products like that thanks to my work in the eating disorder field and to all of my feminist friends. (For the record, a feminist is not someone who hates men and burns bras but someone who believes in the equality of the sexes.) So I said, "No thanks," to the thigh cream, but I left the party wondering about it.

I thought, "Maybe a little thigh cream wouldn't be so bad. After all, I use lipstick. What's the difference?" Then I thought, "Buying thigh cream would make me a hypocrite. I can't talk about loving my body by day and then put on thigh cream by night!"

So I thought and I thought. I'm very good at thinking but not as good at making decisions (which is why this book includes

"What Would Jenni Do?" in Part 6). A week or so after the makeup party, I went to an already-scheduled appointment with my doctor and decided that I would bring up the thigh cream. I asked, "Do thigh creams work?"

"Nope," he said. "I've never seen one that does."

I actually felt relieved. Decision made: I won't buy it.

"But this does," he said and handed me a brochure advertising some type of laser procedure that removes cellulite from your thighs. Instantly, deep down in my gut, I felt something yell, "No!" I even waved my hands and said out loud, "No, no, no!"

Getting a laser procedure to remove cellulite instantly felt wrong to me. I had learned from Carolyn Costin, who is one of my feminist friends, that being recovered means I will not betray my soul to look a certain way. I had worked hard in recovery to learn how to love and respect my body, and taking a laser to my legs did not feel loving or respectful. Instead, it felt like I would be waging war against my body. Another feminist friend, Margo Maine, actually coined the term *body wars* in her revolutionary book of the same name. I had just ended one war against my body that had taken the form of an eating disorder. Did I really want to start another one? Did I really want to invest time and money in removing my cellulite when I had spent so much time and money in therapy learning to embrace it? No and no.

By the time I left my doctor's office that day, I could see clearly that thigh cream—even if it did work—would not be right for me now. I want to devote my time and energy to living and chasing after my dreams—not to chasing after society's ever-changing beauty ideal. The way beauty standards change (a certain physical characteristic is "in," and then it's "out"), cellulite would come "in" just after I had mine removed.

Most people want to look good, and that's okay. But we shouldn't sell our souls or compromise our health in the name of looking good. We cross a line when we betray ourselves just to meet some narrow definition of beauty. If I truly connect with my heart in the moment, I know what feels like a betrayal and what doesn't. To me, wearing makeup feels good as a form of creativity and self-expression. But I admit that it wasn't always this way. Prior to getting into recovery, I felt like I *had* to wear makeup. I wouldn't even walk to the mailbox without it. That was not a form of self-expression; it was a prison.

I chose to keep my cellulite. You might make a different decision based on different reasons, and that's okay. Whether or not we use thigh cream or wear makeup is not the real issue here. The important thing is to look at how we each arrive at our personal decisions. We must look at the why behind what we do. We must be true to ourselves and make choices that are consistent with our beliefs and values.

Today, I wore shorts and felt proud to show off my cellulite. It turns out that it's not so unsightly after all. A lot of people actually did see it, and they still love me. Most important, I still love me.

Real Action: The Beauty Ideal

The beauty ideal is forever changing. We can't keep up! Today's society falsely tells us that the happiest and most successful people are the unrealistically thin ones. Imagine a world where everyone believed that the happiest and most successful people were the ones at their natural weight.

Better yet, imagine a world where being at your natural weight was embraced by society without having to be tied to happiness or success at all. How would your life be different? Take a moment to answer this question.

There's No Place Like Home

ONE, TWO, THREE. I clicked my heels together. I wasn't in the magical land of Oz with Dorothy. I was actually in a voice lesson with my coach, Judy Rodman. (This is the same Judy you read about in *Life Without Ed*, who trapped me in my dietitian's office years ago and forced me to drink a Gatorade—or so it seemed.) Being aware of my heels and clicking them together actually helps me be in tune with my entire body while singing.

When I was lost in my eating disorder, I was disconnected from my body. I felt like a floating head with no body at all. When I sang, I was stiff and rigid like a stick figure. Apparently this is also how I appeared in therapy sessions, because in both my voice lessons and therapy, I was encouraged to move—anything at all. I seemed lifeless.

I used to see my body simply as something to be controlled, but I now see it as a place to live. Like Dorothy says in *The Wizard of Oz*, "There's no place like home."

My friend Dave and I sometimes talk about how we are all just souls in bodies. What body we end up living in while we are on earth is all chance. No matter what body we have—whether we would like it to be taller or shorter—it is where we live, and we must take care of it. Our body is our home.

For more than twenty years, I was at war with my body. I didn't trust it, and for good reason: it didn't trust me. After hard work in recovery and lots of time, after pushing through the pain and not turning back, my body and I are no longer at war. We have called a truce, and we trust each other.

There is nothing like really living in my body. I enjoy experiences today that I used to hate. One example is dancing. I used to like going to school dances, but I dreaded actually dancing. I would go out on the dance floor with my friends and uncomfortably sway back and forth and side to side. I felt awkward, like everyone else was staring at me. Meanwhile, my friends weren't staring at me; they were having fun doing the running man and various break-dancing moves. (It was the early nineties.) I'm comfortable in my body now, and I understand why my friends liked dancing so much. I'm still not an expert at the running man, and I don't have to be to enjoy feeling my body move. I *can* do a pretty good electric slide.

Living in my body also means feeling my feelings on a whole new level. After I recovered, I thought my first broken heart might kill me. The pain was raw and hurt to the core. I remember thinking, "Now I understand why people cry over broken hearts." When I was with Ed, I never had a broken heart, or at least, I never felt it.

The good part about all of this is that now when I feel good, I feel that to the core too. I never knew happiness could be so, well, happy! When I laugh, I feel vibrations deep in my chest, and I usually cry too (happy tears). This never happened before. Living in my body takes life to a whole new dimension. I wouldn't trade it for anything.

Now that I'm living in my body, I can connect more easily on a soul-to-soul level with people around me. I do my best to see others for who they really are on the inside, and they can see the real me too. Interestingly, I've learned that attraction between people is all about this connection. People are attracted to my energy, to my soul, not to my body like I used to think, and that feels good. I have finally discovered peace at home.

Do you have a war going on at home? Maybe it's time to call a truce with your body. Like me and mine, you two will be together for a long time. There really is no place like home. Click your heels together and experience it.

One, two, three!

The Return (Well, Not Really) of the Scale

I HEARD A KNOCK at my door. I opened it to find my friend Sarah standing there holding a bathroom scale. She held out her arms and handed it to me. She said that she had been struggling a lot with her eating disorder and had finally vowed to stop obsessively weighing herself. She wasn't yet ready to toss the scale in the trash, but she was willing to turn it over to me, at least for a while, until she could get rid of it for good.

I shoved the scale into the back of my closet with other things people have given me over the past few years when they're trying to take their power back from Ed. I have a couple of old prom dresses, several pairs of jeans, and one particularly ugly bridesmaid gown. (While it's an aesthetically beautiful dress, I think of it as ugly because I know how much my friend tortured herself to fit into it.)

I had broken the habit of weighing myself years earlier, so I was never tempted to step on the scale Sarah had given me. In fact, I had forgotten about it entirely until my friend Melody picked me up to take me to the airport one day. Looking at my overstuffed suitcase, I said, "I hope this bag isn't too heavy. The airlines only allow up to fifty pounds."

Melody asked, "Let's just weigh it. Do you have a scale?"

I remembered Sarah's and brought it out. The suitcase was too large to balance on the scale by itself without toppling over. So Melody quickly jumped on the scale while holding the bag in her hand. Taking note of the combined weight of herself and the bag, she then put the suitcase down and found her weight alone. Subtracting one number from the other, she said, "Your bag weighs about forty-nine pounds."

I thought to myself, "Wow!"

This was not a wow at Melody's mathematical skills or that my bag would barely make it on the plane, but a wow that she didn't even give a second thought to weighing herself. Melody has never struggled with an eating disorder, and it was glaringly obvious that the scale held no power in her life whatsoever. I thought to myself, "Now that is freedom."

This reminded me of hearing a presentation by my friend and colleague Evelyn Tribole, coauthor of *Intuitive Eating*, at a professional conference about eating disorders a couple of years earlier. Speaking about recovering from weight obsession, she said that recovered people often say, "I'm recovered. I don't even know my weight today."

I was surprised when Evelyn went on to say that even more freedom would be getting to the point of actually being able to know the number on the scale without it mattering—something about being able to get on the scale once, know the number, and then be done with it. I sank back in my chair, thinking, "Yikes! I don't know if I could do that."

At that point in my life, I found incredible peace in not knowing my weight. What I didn't find very peaceful was the fear I experienced in doctors' offices, worrying that someone might accidentally tell me my weight. I worried what might happen if I knew the number. I already told you about the car wreck I had as a result of my gynecologist accidentally spilling the beans. I didn't want to damage myself or any more cars.

Years after hearing Evelyn's presentation and months after witnessing Melody's nonreaction to the scale, I talked with Ann about weighing myself. We both agreed that the return of the scale—just to get on it once—might actually be helpful to me. So without hesitation, I stepped on the scale and looked at the number. Nothing.

No, I didn't weigh nothing. *Nothing* as in no energy, no emotion. Just a number. Another wow! I haven't weighed myself since.

(You'll be glad to know that Sarah eventually threw the scale out.) I am no longer scared to accidentally hear my weight in the doctor's office. Just when I thought I couldn't feel any freer, I do!

If I had stepped on the scale before this, I might have had an entirely different reaction, possibly a bad one. For many years, finding out my weight wasn't worth the risk of possibly losing the freedom I gained by not knowing it. If you think you want to step on the scale, talk with your treatment team about your motives behind that desire. Some recovered people might choose never to know their weight, and that's okay. All of our paths are different.

I still don't weigh myself, but I know my approximate weight. The difference between what Ed wanted me to weigh and what I weigh now is many pounds of happiness. That is weight I never want to lose. No *weigh*!

NOTE TO ED: If you're reading this, Ed, don't use this section to get people who are better off not knowing their weight to find it out. I'm on to you and your tactics. Oh, and Ed, the reader is on to you too.

Real Action: What's Holding You Back?

What are you holding on to that keeps you stuck in weight obsession—a scale, specific clothes, or something else entirely? Do your best to get rid of these things. If you have a strong inner resistance to tossing something specific, this is probably something you most need to give up. If you can't commit to giving something up entirely, ask a friend to watch over it for a while and promise to give it back when you want it. My guess is that you'll find life much better without whatever it is.

If you do have to get rid of some clothes, go a step further and buy new, healthy ones. Go shopping with a friend or family member and have him or her help you select clothes without letting you see the sizes. After buying the clothes, have your shopping buddy cut out all of the size tags. You will have sizeless clothes in a sizeless closet. I did this with my mom years ago, and it helped a lot. (Today, I don't have to ask someone to remove size tags when I go shopping because, like the scale, clothes no longer hold power over me.)

6

THE PERFECTLY IMPERFECT WEDDING

Overcoming Perfectionism

No wedding can be perfect. No marriage—to yourself or anyone else—can be perfect. To leave my eating disorder behind and find true joy in life, I had to tackle my perfectionism with the same intensity I had used with Ed. I had to look at my tendency to be rigid and practice being more flexible, even if it meant being less than (or far from) perfect. Whether you struggle with a high level of perfectionism like I did or battle it to a lesser degree, Part 6 will help you take some steps toward more happiness in this perfectly imperfect life.

This Book

THIS BOOK—APPROXIMATELY SIXTY thousand words arranged in a sensible order—is due to my publisher in twenty-four hours. Even though I'm not yet finished writing, I just went out and had a long, relaxing dinner with a friend. (Yes, going out to eat *is* relaxing.) Earlier today, I had coffee with another friend just to laugh and have fun. Last weekend, I went hiking and saw a movie with another friend. Over the past week, I have been focusing lots of energy (probably too much) on a guy I like—instant messaging, texting, and mostly just wondering if he'll call.

I'm writing this book—it will be turned in on time—and I didn't have to be a perfectionistic workaholic to get it done. I didn't work nonstop. I didn't lose sleep. In fact, I had more fun than ever.

Don't get me wrong. I am far from being perfect at dealing with perfectionism, but now I know that progress, not perfection, is the goal. While I still have to deal with it on some level, I get better all the time, and I'm light-years away from where I used to be. Light-years upon light-years. (That might sound a little perfectionistic. I told you I still have to work at it.) But the fact that you're reading this book, that I actually finished it, is proof of my progress.

I didn't write this book for a long time (you read about my varying excuses in "A Different Decision," in Part 2) because I was scared that it wouldn't be as good as my first book. A publisher (not mine) told me that an author's second book is a perceived failure, so I put off writing this one—my second—and then I put it off some more. If I didn't write it, it couldn't be a failure. What was really going on was perfectionism, and as it often does, it led to procrastination and a lack of productivity.

After I finally began to write the book (a deadline always helps to kick-start the process), I struggled with how I was going to fit more than five years' worth of information—therapy work, professional conference notes, personal journals, and more—into one manuscript. As I wrote, I would hit a standstill, feel overwhelmed, and think that I would never have enough time to sort through all of this information. The draft is due in one day, and guess who still has piles and piles of unread, not-yet-looked-through material?

What I have realized in writing this book is that what I have to say doesn't come from something I jotted down in a therapy session last week or at a professional conference two years ago. No, my message comes straight from my heart. It is real, not perfect.

My last hurdle in getting the draft finished has been this section on perfectionism. Interestingly enough, I caught myself wanting the part on perfectionism to be, well, perfect. I was spinning my wheels trying to write about every way to tackle perfectionism that I have ever learned in therapy and life. I ultimately realized that I could only talk authentically about what has worked for me, so that's what you'll find here. Everything I write about might not work for you, but as with everything else, take what is helpful and leave the rest.

So this is the first short section about perfectionism. It's not perfect, but, of course, it doesn't have to be. I did my best with integrity, and that is all I can ever do. After reading Part 6, my hope is that you might be closer to realizing that the same is true for you.

A New Motivator

I STAYED IN BED all day long. I felt paralyzed. I felt depressed. This was one of those low points where I knew I would feel at least a little better if I picked up the phone and called someone. But the phone was just too far away—two steps too far away. I couldn't pull together that much energy. I had a headache, my stomach hurt, and I had thrown up earlier. You might be surprised, but this wasn't about Ed. It was about perfectionism.

I had been free from destructive behaviors with food for a significant period. I had thrown up not to get rid of calories but because my stomach was turning in circles from anxiety and worry. I wasn't accomplishing anything because I was trying to be perfect at everything. Well, maybe not *everything*. I no longer obsessed about food and weight, but there was still everything else.

This is part of what kept me in bed that day. In a world where it's not possible to be perfect at everything, Ed had promised that I could always be perfect at one thing. Even if everything else in my life slipped away or was imperfect, I could be the perfect weight according to Ed. I could control what I ate even if I could not control other things. With Ed gone, this sense of control was gone. He had been a buffer to my perfectionistic tendencies, and without my buffer, I felt them full force.

Ed had always promised relief from the anxiety and stress of perfectionism through restricting, bingeing, and purging. Without him, I didn't know how to cope. I felt the pain of perfectionism more than ever, but I still chased after it. I just couldn't stop chasing the mirage, even though I could never get there. If I got a raise at work, I should have gotten a bigger one. If I got a bigger one, I should have gotten it sooner. I couldn't win and felt beaten down most of the time.

I wondered why I had worked so hard to recover from my eating disorder only to feel this bad. As things went downhill, I began to wonder which was worse—Ed or perfectionism. Sometimes it seemed like I was lower than ever.

Lying in my bed that day, I was at yet another crossroads. Perfectionism would push me back into Ed's arms for relief (and I might die with him the next time around), or I would continue to live in a miserable state that was getting worse every day. I also thought that this might kill me. While I never wanted to kill myself, I thought about "not existing" a lot. For instance, I would be driving on a highway overpass and think, "It wouldn't bother me if my car accidentally flew off the overpass right now and crashed into the moving cars below." When would I finally commit to doing whatever it took to recover from my perfectionism?

My treatment team had tried to convince me for years to face perfectionism head-on. They said that perfectionism was just as toxic for me as bingeing (or acting out with some other eating disordered behavior), but I just didn't believe that it was that big a problem. I thought that a life without eating disordered behaviors was all I needed, and I actually credited perfectionism with all of my accomplishments. If I didn't hold on to perfectionism as my motivator in life, I didn't think I would be motivated to do anything. My team said I needed a new motivator. I thought they just wanted to make me lazy, just as during eating disorder recovery, I had thought they just wanted to make me fat. (I was wrong on both counts.)

Without perfectionism as my motivator, I thought I would just be lying around all day doing nothing. Yet there I was at rock bottom with my perfectionism, and what was I doing? *Lying around all day doing nothing.* Perfectionism had strangely created the same situation I had been trying to avoid. Was I finally convinced?

Yes, I knew I had to change. I had to find other ways to achieve my goals. Although perfectionism had pushed me to get things done for a while, I had paid a high price. It stole my joy. It negatively impacted my spirituality by telling me that praying and other spiritual pursuits were unproductive. Perfectionism led to my looking at life with a pessimistic attitude instead of gratitude. It led to scarcity thinking, saying there wasn't enough for everyone, so I needed to act first, and I needed to be stronger and better than anyone else. Using perfection as a motivator disconnected me from everyone else and ran me into the ground.

It took time and patience (and lots of therapy) to get off the ground, but I finally connected with a new motivator, a deep, peaceful, and joyful place inside—my heart. Connecting with my heart rather than perfectionism was another one of those "jumping" points in life (see "Jump," in Part 2). I had to let go, have faith, and trust.

Knowing what's best for me, my heart does not drive me to reach impossible standards. Unlike perfectionism, which causes me to ignore or discount what I have achieved, my heart fully acknowledges my accomplishments. It provides me with the self-confidence to move forward in a healthy way.

My eating disorder and perfectionism worked together, strengthened each another, to hold me down. The cool thing is that recovery from my eating disorder and recovery from my perfectionism also strengthen each other to lift me up. In recovering from both an eating disorder and perfectionism, the whole is greater than the sum of its parts. It's synergy. Perfectionism—adhering to mathematical rules—tells me that one plus one always equals two, but I know—I am living proof—how one (eating disorder recovery) plus one (recovery from perfectionism) can equal much, much more.

Real Action: The Truth About Perfectionism

Society tells us to be perfect. You and I both know the truth about that. It's impossible. In therapy, I made two lists in my journal about the advantages and disadvantages of perfectionism. Here are a few examples:

Benefits of Perfectionism
- High productivity
- Good grades and awards
- Impressive résumé

 ### Negative Consequences of Perfectionism
- Low to no spirituality
- No close friends
- No joy in life

Make two lists of your own. You will discover that any gains from perfectionism are not worth the losses. You will also realize that the benefits only last for so long. Running your life on perfectionism is like running your car on dirty gasoline; it might go but not for long (and not as efficiently). If you're like me, you might also discover that you can actually achieve many of the items on your benefits list in a healthy, balanced way. Looking at my list, for example, I'm a lot more productive (and more balanced) in the long run by connecting with my heart rather than perfectionism.

Good Enough

"THAT'S GOOD ENOUGH," my friends in school used to say as they hurriedly finished their homework assignments at the last minute. Well, *good enough* wasn't good enough for me. I would think to myself, "They don't have to be perfect, but I do." I held myself—but not others—to an unrealistic ideal. Today I know that double standards like this usually mean I'm not making much sense.

My goal of perfection seemed attainable when I was a student in school—living within the simplistic measurement system of grades. If I didn't miss a question on a test, I did perfectly. As long as I had tests to take and homework to complete, I could live within the illusion of perfection. No matter what else was going on in my life—good, bad, or indifferent—I could prevail as the perfect student.

After college, I no longer received a regular report card listing a string of As to tell me I was perfect. The real world is not as simple as As, Bs, and Cs. It is subjective, complicated, and messy. Perfection doesn't exist in the real world, only perfectionism does.

Overcoming perfectionism means challenging black-and-white thinking and opening up to the gray area. In the past, my brain could only compute perfection or failure—nothing in between. So words like *competent, acceptable, satisfactory,* and *good enough* fell into the failure category. Even *above average* meant failure. If I received an 88 out of 100 percent on an exam, I felt that I failed. The fact is most things in life are not absolutes and have components of both good and bad.

I used to think in absolute terms a lot: *all, every,* or *never.* I would eat all of the food (that is, binge), and then I would vow to restrict every meal and to never eat again. This type of thinking extended outside of the food arena as well: I had to get all of the answers right on a test; I had to be in every extracurricular activity; if I didn't make the school's highest-ranking volleyball team, I would never play again. Well, I didn't make that team once, so I didn't play any more volleyball in school. The "if it's not perfect, I quit" approach to life is a treacherous way to live.

As a writer, I used to think that everything I wrote was either absolutely wonderful or completely awful. The truth is that sometimes what I write isn't on a par with Shakespeare, but it's still good. I could never recognize this before, because I hadn't established a baseline of competence: What gets the job done? What is *good enough*?

Finding good enough takes trial and error. For those of us who are perfectionists, the *error* part of trial and error can stop us dead in our tracks. We would rather keep chasing perfection than risk possibly making a mistake. I was able to change my behavior only when the pain of perfectionism became greater that the pain of making an error. (I don't believe that we always have to get to the point of extreme pain before making changes. It does seem to be my pattern though. I'm working on that.)

Today good enough means that I'm okay just the way I am. I play my position in the world. I catch the ball when it is thrown my way. I don't always have to make the crowd go wild or get a standing ovation. It's good enough to just catch the ball or even to do my best to catch it. Good enough means that I finally enjoy playing the game.

To my surprise, the good enough solution is often even more effective than the perfect solution. Always trying to find the perfect answer slows you down and can even stop you completely. You get so caught up in the details that you miss the big picture. The good enough solution frees up more time and energy for what really matters in your life. In my life, I have more time to spend with people close to me, more time to laugh, more time to live.

Today I can truly say, "That's good enough."

Real Action: Perfectly Imperfect Reminders

When I was looking for good enough, it helped to leave perfectly imperfect reminders throughout my life. Some examples are lopsided window shades in my living room, a coffee stain on my car seat, and a hole in my sock.

I didn't purposely hang my shades crooked, but after spending an unusually long time trying to hang them "just right," I finally stopped and accepted that imperfect is okay. Even today, when I see my shades, I remember that I've been doing all right even though the shades are not exactly right.

The next time you find yourself getting caught up trying to do something perfectly, take a moment to breathe—and then walk away. Create a perfectly imperfect reminder for yourself. If this is helpful, do it again and again.

What Scares Me Most
About Growing Up

*W*HAT SCARES ME *most about being a full-grown,*
healthy adult is not being successful. As long as I am not
a full-grown, healthy adult, I don't have to do everything right.
I still have room to grow, to become a success. If I am not full-
grown and healthy, nothing is set in stone. There is still time.

I'm still growing. I don't have to be perfect yet.

The above excerpt is from a journal entry I wrote during early recovery. I was answering a question posed in therapy: "What scares you most about being a full-grown, healthy adult?"

Staying in my eating disorder kept me a kid. It kept me dependent on others financially and emotionally. It gave me excuses for why I didn't have a "real" job and why I couldn't pursue this or that. I once said, "I can't pursue music right now, because I'm too sick." At certain points along the way, I really was too sick to pursue music. What I needed to do during those times was focus on recovery and become willing to do whatever it took to get better. I didn't do this for a long time, because part of me liked having the eating disorder as an excuse. As long as I had Ed, I was a person who had never pursued music instead of one who had pursued music and failed. Today I'm finally getting back on track with my music efforts.

Ed gave me the same kind of excuse for not being in dating relationships. I told many men, "I can't date you. I'm too sick."

Again, maybe I really was too sick to date. I should have used this as motivation to recover, but instead I used it as motivation to stay sick and get out of dating.

On the opposite side of the coin, I sometimes used being sick as a tactic to get a man (or someone else) to take care of me, to love me. They might love me if I were sick, but would they love me if I were well? I have since learned I don't have to be sick to be loved.

As long as I had an eating disorder, I thought people couldn't expect me to have it all together. They couldn't expect me to be perfect. But if I got better, they could—and would—expect perfection. I thought I'd better stay sick to avoid those high expectations. (I eventually figured out it wasn't they who had the high expectations, but me.)

I thought I'd better stay sick to avoid becoming a woman too. You see, I wasn't just scared of growing up; I was also specifically afraid of becoming a woman. In middle school, I remember hoping I would never begin menstruating. My classmates actually made fun of girls and looked down on them for getting their period. I often wonder what it would have been like if we had celebrated menstruation and looked at it as something exciting instead. Today I have heard people talk about menstruation ceremonies that do just that.

I was scared to have curves and to wear a bra. Ed said, "You might have to become a woman, but you don't have to look like one." If I didn't look like a woman, I still felt like a little girl on the inside. This feeling was safe and familiar. I was still daddy's little girl, and I didn't have to take on the responsibilities of an adult. A big problem was that I never voiced these fears to anyone, not until I got into recovery from my eating disorder.

In therapy, I learned that my definition of success needed to change radically. In my world, failure was a very broad category. My successful category was so small that it was impossible for me—or anyone else—to fit into it. To be successful, I had to be perfect in the world's eyes. This included having the rail-thin, hipless body of a little girl.

At first, I thought changing my definition of success would just be an excuse to be lazy and mediocre. Now I see the truth. I had to change my definition of success to live a full life. I learned that true success is not having a prosperous career or a curveless body. Success, like happiness, comes from the inside. Success is living in the moment and feeling joy. It's living in a healthy woman's body.

The other day, I parked my rental car at a hotel, and the GPS navigation system said, "You have arrived." I laughed, because I knew that I might have arrived at my destination in the parking lot, but I have not arrived in life. Like everyone else, I'm still a work in progress. We never arrive. Like my journal entry says, "I'm still growing." I never have to be perfect.

Making Waves

I USED TO LIVE by the motto "Don't make waves." I did my best not to cause problems or upset anyone. I was nearly perfect at not rocking the proverbial boat.

The not-so-perfect thing was that, in order not to make waves, I had to sit on the shore while others seemed to be having fun in the water. You cannot move through water without making a wake. You can't even put one foot in without making some ripples. Since I was afraid to make even the smallest of waves, I was stuck.

I stayed on the shore worrying about what everyone else thought of me. I was stuck trying to please all and disappoint none. The only person I didn't take into account was myself.

A large part of my eating disorder actually revolved around this approval seeking. Most obvious, I wanted to be thin to get society's approval. Less apparent but even more significant, my eating disorder actually became a coping mechanism for my people-pleasing behaviors. I dealt with my almost constant state of anger and resentment (a common result of people pleasing) by bingeing, purging, and restricting. Long after Ed and I divorced, the people pleasing stuck around. Sooner or later, I knew this behavior would lead me back to Ed, so I needed to change.

In Twelve Step meetings for my eating disorder, I had often heard, "What other people think of me is none of my business." My job is not to worry about what everyone else thinks about me but to discover what I think. If I actually want to know what someone else thinks, my job is then to ask that person. More often than not, however, it isn't important to know. It's okay if people are mad at me, and it's okay if people think I'm a complete idiot—as long as I'm doing my best. Just because certain people might have judgments about me, it does not mean they have authority over me.

To truly own my own life, I had to ask questions like "What are my needs?" and "What are my thoughts?" I had to acknowledge both my strengths and my weaknesses. I had to form my own opinions based on my reality instead of someone else's.

In the beginning, I just tested the waters, put my little toe in to make some ripples. I stopped sending greeting cards to every person I know for every occasion. To take care of my needs, I sometimes missed other people's birthdays and anniversaries. I'm not sure anyone even noticed (except Hallmark). I stopped answering every e-mail and phone call.

Over time, I actually walked into the water and made some small waves. I began expressing my true desires by speaking clearly and concisely. First, I practiced with people I trusted, including my friends, family, and therapist. I learned that "No" is a complete sentence. In other words, when I say no to someone, I don't need to provide a long, drawn-out explanation of why I said it. While an explanation can be important in certain instances, most of the time saying more just leads to overexplaining that is neither helpful nor necessary. On the opposite end of the spectrum, I learned that sometimes I needed to say yes (as in "Yes, I do need help").

Recently I made a big wave. For the first time in as long as I can remember, I missed a deadline for a project. I forgot about the Monday deadline because I was having so much fun over the weekend with friends. (Being irresponsible is actually progress for me!) I had always thought that missing a deadline would make a tsunami-like wave. To my surprise, the resulting waves didn't have as much power as I expected. Even more shocking to me, people can actually go with the flow and ride the waves.

All I can ever do is my best in any given moment. And my best varies depending on the moment. Sometimes my best means that I need to get some much-needed rest and relaxation—and miss someone else's deadline. For the most part, when I get my needs met, I am better at genuinely meeting other people's needs without feeling resentful.

Today I love being out in the water. I'm not afraid to rock the boat when I need to, and I don't panic when I rock a boat by accident. Sometimes my actions upset people; sometimes I make mistakes and disappoint others. If you live your entire life without ever disappointing anyone, you're not living.

Put on your swimsuit (another topic altogether; see "Are You a Prisoner?" in Part 5), splash around, and start making waves!

Real Action: Make Waves of Your Own

When I first began making waves in my life, I actually rocked some boats (small ones) on purpose to practice experiencing the uncomfortable feelings and help build my confidence that these actions really were okay.

The first boat I rocked involved sending e-mail. I used to spend an inordinate amount of time rereading each and every e-mail I wrote for mistakes before I sent it out into cyberspace. I spell-checked messages at least once, and sometimes two or three times.

While sometimes it's important to check thoroughly for mistakes before sending an e-mail (for business correspondence), most of the time it's okay to glance over it quickly (or not at all) and just hit Send. This gets the job done and saves time.

To get to this point, I first began sending e-mails without spell-checking. Time and again, I would realize that I had sent something with a misspelled word, and time and again, it didn't seem to matter. Then I purposely began to send e-mails that I knew were not exactly right. The wording was messed up in some way, or the punctuation was off. I would hit Send, and it still didn't seem to make a difference in my goals, personally or professionally (and I'm a writer). The only difference, and it was a good one, is that my time was freed up to do things aside from e-mail.

I challenge you to make a wave by sending an imperfect e-mail or two. You can even send one to me if you want. Begin to see how people in your life can ride the waves of incorrect spelling and punctuation. See how much more fun you have out in the water!

Will You Run in the Waterfall?

MY FIRST-GRADE TEACHER wrote my name on the chalk-board for talking in class. She had very strict rules about when we could and could not talk. I had broken a rule, and I had to pay the consequence by getting my name written on the board. I cried and cried, then I cried some more until, out of desperation to get me to stop, she finally erased my name. I stopped crying and vowed never to break another rule in school.

I never got my name on the board again. Instead, each year, I got more and more in touch with inflexibility and perfectionism. Rules ruled my life. This rigidity would eventually become a big part of my eating disorder. Ed has rules for everything, he thrives on them, and he says we shouldn't break them—or else. When we finally get strong enough to break Ed's rules, we realize "or else" actually means that we experience an amazingly happy life. It also means that we are prepared to face the next phase of personal growth work, which for me, in part, meant challenging rigidity in other areas of my life.

I no longer follow any of Ed's directives, but I still put too much emphasis on rules in general, any rule. And if there isn't a rule for something, I'm quite talented at inventing one. Recently, I created a rule while on a day hike with a group of people. At one point along the trail, several of the hikers ran in a waterfall and started splashing around in the water. I wanted to go in too, but I initially stopped myself, thinking, "What if I'm not supposed to run in the waterfall? What if the hike leader gets mad at us for playing in the water?"

Thanks to my newfound awareness of my rigidity, I realized that I was probably making up another rule that didn't exist—a

"Do not play in a waterfall" rule. Eventually, I decided to run in the waterfall with everyone else, including the hike leader.

I tried to make up that rule in the middle of the woods because I have always felt more comfortable in well-structured environments that have rules. I think that's why Ed had such a great hold on me for so long.

I functioned very well within the dictates of the school system. After college, I actually liked the rules associated with working in a restaurant or an office. Clocking in, clocking out, and even the various dress codes felt comfortable to me.

I struggle today with the fact that I have a job that gives me tremendous freedom. As a self-employed person, I don't have to clock in or clock out. There is no dress code in my home office. I can wear my favorite pink pajamas to work every day. While I do love this flexibility, it can also be scary at times.

I don't have a boss, but I keep trying to give myself rules, regulations, and requirements. Just the other day, I asked my friend Rob, who is also self-employed, "How many hours is a person supposed to work during the week?"

Rob said, "There are no rules." He explained that he functions best when he works a certain number of hours per week, and that the number changes depending on the project he is working on at the time and just how he feels in general.

I had wanted Rob to give me some specific rule about the number of hours I should be working. If he had given me a rule, I could easily have followed it and felt comfortable. If he had said that I should work thirty-two hours, thirty-five minutes, and two seconds each week, I could have done that. Simple. Instead, he told me that I have to decide what works best for me at each specific time in my life. Not as easy to figure out.

The older I get, the more I realize that there often are no rules. There are guidelines and recommendations, like how many hours to sleep per night or how much money to spend on your first house, but we each have to decide for ourselves what fits us best. I work daily on being more flexible and breaking out of my little rule-shaped box.

I also work hard to determine which of my rules actually help me. I've realized that sometimes, instead of breaking out of my box, I need to stay within that safety zone in order to take care of myself. For instance, certain personal rules related to dating work for me. I'm learning what works through trial and error (aka making mistakes).

There are no rules about which rules to follow, which ones to break, which ones to shatter, and which ones don't even exist.

If I get my name on the chalkboard today, I won't cry. I will know that I'm following my own compass and walking to the beat of my own drum. Will you dare to get your name on the chalkboard? Will you run in the waterfall?

If It Can Be Done, It Must Be Done

I KNEW I WAS making tremendous progress in my recovery from perfectionism when I stopped reading a book midway through. I didn't like the book, so I didn't finish it. And I felt awful. As an active member of the If It Can Be Done, It Must Be Done program, I also believed, "If it can be read, it must be read." I had spent hours and hours reading books I didn't like just to finish them. Unfinished books made me feel anxious.

If it can be done, it must be done. This used to be my philosophy for life. In high school, if I *could* take all advanced placement (AP) and honors classes, I *had to* take all AP and honors classes. If I *could* get straight As, I *had to* get straight As. As I got older and joined the real world, if something came across my desk, it had to be done. If an e-mail entered my Inbox, I had to respond to it. If I could pick my friend up from the airport, I had to.

If you try to do everything that comes your way like this, there is no time left over for rest and relaxation, for rejuvenation. Yes, in school, I was capable of making straight As, and I did. But now I can see that getting good grades at the expense of my health and happiness wasn't worth it. Some eating disorder treatment programs actually require certain patients to get at least one B (instead of all As) each semester. Many patients are encouraged not to take all AP or honors classes. To recover, we have to simplify our lives.

Throughout my recovery, I learned how to set limits and prioritize. Not only did I used to think I had to do everything that came across my desk, but I also believed that everything was top priority. Everything can't be number one, and believing this is setting yourself up for unhappiness. I learned how to prioritize. In the beginning, for simplicity's sake (and to avoid getting absorbed in some complicated, perfectionistic system, which I've been known to do), I just prioritized things that came across my desk into three categories: very important, important, and not important. Almost all of the items that fell into the not important category never got done, and many of the items in the other two categories never got done either. Just because something can be done doesn't mean that it has to be done.

Everyone has a limited amount of time and energy, so in therapy, I learned to think about energy efficiency. I accepted that each day only includes twenty-four hours, and I have to make time for what matters most. I've learned that I can't possibly do everything that comes my way and also be happy. I can do a lot of it (still, probably not all) and be miserable and depressed; I lived like this for years, and I won't do it any longer.

Today I'm content if I do A or B or C in a day. I no longer have to do A and B and C. Sometimes I do D or nothing at all, and that's okay too. My recovered life leaves room for such spontaneity. As I sit here writing, I see several unfinished books scattered throughout my home. I'm just fine with that.

Perfectionism might be telling you that you have to finish this book just because you started it. You don't. You don't even have to finish this paragraph if you don't want to. And I don't have to finish writing this sen . . .

What Would Jenni Do?

I WAS HAVING COFFEE with my friend Dave recently and asked him what I should do about this guy, about that situation, and about something else too. I think I have a bad habit of asking Dave, "What would you do?" because this time he paused, looked me in the eye, and said, "What would Jenni do?" He told me I needed to start trusting myself more.

It's funny that he said that, because Ann had just told me that I needed to begin "trusting me with me" more. It's okay to get other people's opinions, but in the end, I need to trust my own judgment. Other people don't have my answers. All signs point to the fact that I'm a grown, healthy adult who can make my own decisions.

My difficulty with making decisions began a long time ago. For many years, Ed made a lot of my decisions, both small and big. You can imagine that he decided what I ate, what I wore, and how I treated my body, but he also called the shots in other areas. If I couldn't decide whether or not to go to a party, he would say, "Let's binge tonight." Decision made. I would binge and not go to the party. If the party ended up being fabulous, I would think, "It's not my fault I missed out on a great party. Ed made me stay home."

Ed also made my decisions related to dating and sexuality. He decided that he would be the only man in my life. In this way and others, he seemed to simplify things for me. With Ed in charge, life—with its endless questions and possibilities—seemed small and manageable. Sometimes I felt as if I were walking around in a trancelike state. All I had to think about was food and weight. Of course, we all know that life was really unmanageable with Ed running the show. This unmanageability drove me to get professional help for my eating disorder.

My treatment team asked me to hand some of the power I had given Ed over to them for a while. My internist was in charge of my weight; my dietitian was in charge of what I ate. Because my eating disorder was about a lot more than just weight and food, my team provided guidance to me in other areas as well. The problem became that I didn't want them just to guide me in specific areas. I wanted them to tell me exactly what to do in all areas. Even after I had been in recovery for a significant amount of time, I would still ask my team to make decisions for me. They would say, "Jenni, we can't decide that for you."

This reminded me a lot of my parents. As I grew up, they had wanted me to make more and more decisions on my own and would often say, "Jenni, we can't decide that for you."

I was frustrated that my treatment team had received the same memo my parents had been given years earlier. I felt like people were abandoning me when they refused to tell me what to do. In reality, they were empowering me.

Making decisions on my own terrified me. If I made the decision, then the consequences of that decision would lie squarely on my shoulders. I couldn't blame anyone else when things went wrong.

To overcome this fear of doing the wrong thing, my team encouraged me to simply practice being decisive instead of being right. Naturally, I didn't apply this theory to questions about food and weight. It was still too early in recovery for that. I practiced being decisive when it came to other aspects of my life, questions like "Should I buy the blue or green shirt? Should I move into the downstairs or upstairs apartment? Should I ask for time off work on Thursday or Friday?" Decisions like these used to take an unrealistic amount of time and also send me into tailspins of frustration and worry. When it came to things like this, I simply needed to start making decisions and quit worrying so much about making the right or wrong ones. My motto became "Be decisive."

I was encouraged to get in touch with my true desires when making a decision. When someone asked me a question, I would repeat the question to myself. For example, if someone asked, "Do you want to go to the party?" I repeated, "Do I want to go to the party?" I learned that Ed and other voices in my head would answer the various questions. But over time I began to hear Jenni answer the same question too. I learned that Jenni was the decision maker and had the final say.

In the end, I was surprised to discover that there are usually many right answers to one question. Since there is rarely a perfect answer, I stopped working so hard to find it all the time. Instead of making the "right" decision, I try to make the best decision I can with the information I have. I try to make authentic choices that are not based on shame or fear, but on what I honestly think and feel in the present moment. As I said earlier (see "My Heart," in Part 1), I make my best decisions when I connect with my heart.

I've made a lot of progress in decision making. But life is all about continual growth, and I still have some work to do in this area. I will keep asking, "What would Jenni do?"

More important, I will keep answering. Right or wrong!

Real Action: What Do *You* Want?

Practice making decisions and trusting you with you. Write down three things you know you want. Make sure they are things you *really* want rather than things you *should* want.

1. _____
2. _____
3. _____

Now list three things you know you don't want. Again, make them things you *really* don't want rather than things you *shouldn't* want.

1. _____
2. _____
3. _____

Be decisive. Don't worry about finding the right answer; instead, find the right answers for you.

Having Fun to Save My Life

I WAS PRESCRIBED THIRTY minutes of fun per day. Ann wrote this prescription a few years ago after she heard me say that my idea of fun was folding laundry while simultaneously watching CMT (Country Music Television). I explained to Ann that having something productive to do while watching television—which I considered unproductive through the lens of perfectionism—somehow made the act of watching television permissible. With perfectionism, there was no time for having fun just for the fun of it. Fun could only be tolerated if it were combined with some type of work activity.

I had been assigned fun many years prior during treatment for my eating disorder. At that point, I was actually assigned to watch the television show *Friends* once a week. I remember sitting on my couch, watching the show, and laughing, while feeling extremely guilty at the same time. (Yes, this is the positive kind of guilt that signaled I was moving forward.) At this point, having fun wasn't much fun at all. In fact, it was so painful and exhausting that I ultimately hit a standstill. I had made some progress, but I needed to go further.

This time around, with Ann, I knew I had to make some drastic changes in the fun department, changes that would last a lifetime. I was beginning to see that I couldn't live another thirty years working so much and relaxing so little—I was setting myself up for a heart attack by age thirty-five. I had to have fun to save my life.

Finding the right balance between work and play has been important and challenging. In the beginning, I had to be assigned fun homework in therapy, or I wouldn't have done it. In addition to being prescribed thirty minutes of fun per day, I was once assigned to read a book of fiction. It couldn't be something that I would learn from, such as historical fiction or even sci-fi. It had to be read for fun only. Of course, like before, this wasn't much fun at all. But unlike before, I stuck with the uncomfortable feelings and kept moving forward to the other side.

As I began to strike my own unique balance of fun in my life, I asked Ann questions like, "How much fun should someone my age be having?" and "Is it okay if I go out with friends every night this week to have fun?" Ann knew that I had to find these answers for myself, so she would encourage me to experiment. She would say, "Go out every night this week and see how that feels."

After years of practice and patience, having fun has become more intuitive for me, just like eating and exercise. I know when I need food, when I need exercise, and when I need fun. And I don't feel guilty for enjoying myself anymore, just like I don't feel guilty for eating and exercising in a balanced way.

In addition to seeking out activities just for fun (like going to a concert), I have also learned how to find enjoyment in everything I do. Responding to e-mails for work and even sitting in the airport can be fun. It turns out that fun and work are not separate; they go together. It's all about my attitude.

My attitude has changed for the better. I have choices now. I can choose to have fun folding laundry while watching Carrie Underwood on CMT, or I can choose to put down the laundry basket and go see her perform live.

Won't you come out and play with me? Come on, it'll be fun!

Real Action: Fun for You

I used to feel anxious about having fun and feeling good. Sometimes I even felt like an imposter—like I wasn't really being myself. Well-respected body-image expert Adrienne Ressler, LMSW, says that we experience this anxiety not because we are not being our authentic selves but because feeling good feels so unfamiliar. We have been with Ed for so long that feeling bad actually feels normal. Sometimes what is familiar—even if it is destructive—can feel safe and comfortable to us. To recover, we have to be willing to get uncomfortable:

Plan for one especially fun activity in your schedule this week. Like me, you might find that having fun is not too much fun at first. With practice, it will be. So start practicing!

Along the way, talk with your therapist about any anxiety that you may experience.

7

HAPPILY MARRIED

Falling in Love with Life

I'm not alone anymore. I finally have someone special in my life to stand by my side each day, to lean on during difficult times, and to love me unconditionally. That person is me. Divorcing Ed, the most difficult experience I've ever been through, has brought about the most powerful experience: falling in love with life. One true gift of my recovery has been that I can apply what I've learned along the way to my life today. No longer Ed's bride, I'm married to me. I love me. Part 7 will help you commit to becoming fully recovered and to finding that someone special in your life. You!

Marrying Myself

A COUPLE WEEKS AGO I heard that my ex-fiancé, Mark, had moved on. He had gotten married and moved away. While I was genuinely happy for him, at the same time, I felt a little sad that—more than three years after the breakup—I'm still very single. I asked myself, "Why am I still single while he has moved on?"

I also felt relief that the "Mark" chapter of my life is finally closed. Any buried hope I had of him appearing on my doorstep and promising to do anything to be with me is not going to happen. Even though I knew deep inside that I wouldn't go back to him anyway, I still pictured a more dramatic ending to our relationship—something with a little more Hollywood pizzazz. Now my ties to Mark are severed (pizzazz or not), and I can officially move on. Or might it be possible that I have *already*?

I might not be in a serious dating relationship, and I might not have a ring on my finger, but I have definitely moved on—in much bigger ways than any wedding band could signify. Getting married would have been the easy path for me a few years ago. I chose not to get stuck in a bad relationship but to move forward. That meant being single longer.

Since the day I gave back the engagement ring, I truly started taking my life back in ways that I never thought were possible. I have moved from being in recovery from an eating disorder to being fully recovered. I respect my body and give it what it needs, which includes not only food but also rest, relaxation, and fun. I respect my emotions, allowing myself to feel sad and lonely. I understand that nobody is perfect and celebrate my imperfections. I realize the importance of connecting with God and devote time to that daily.

I'm a different person today than the girl who would have married Mark. I'm no longer a child; I'm proud to finally proclaim that I'm a woman. That scared little girl was not ready to be married and wouldn't have been a very good partner. At that point in my life, I still needed to focus on me. I needed to learn how to truly love myself. I thought I already did, and I had certainly made significant progress in that area, but I still had a lot of personal growth work ahead. Part of that work was realizing that I didn't even want to be married.

Today I'm married to someone I trust, love, honor, and respect, someone who will never leave me—myself! I'm the only person who will always be with me, literally, so this relationship needs to be strong. More than that, I need to cherish and embrace that relationship. I need to get excited about it.

I was going to write a song for Mark's and my wedding, but I never had the chance. Instead, I decided to write something for my marriage to me. Here are my wedding vows:

I, Jenni, take you, Jenni, to be my beautiful bride. Before God, my family, and friends, I promise to cherish you and be true to you in good times and in bad, in sickness and in health. I will love and honor you all the days of my life. I will accept all of your faults and strengths with patience and gentle kindness. I will help you to meet your needs—emotionally, physically, and spiritually. I will watch a funny movie with you when you need to laugh. I will feed you when you are hungry and give you rest when you are tired. I will help you to nourish your relationship with God. I will not leave you again. You never left me. I love you, Jenni.

The best thing about these vows is that I can renew them every day without a white dress or a veil. I can even edit them when I'm working on a particular issue in my life.

I'm going to send these vows to people I trust to make myself accountable. These people would have made the effort to attend my big Texas wedding, so I know they will have time to read a quick message. No need for wedding gifts this time (even though I never did get that set of matching dishes)—all I really need is lots of love and support. I know I already have that from these folks.

Now I have it from me too.

Real Action: Writing Your Vows

Write wedding vows to yourself. Share what you write with trusted people in your life. Post your vows in your home somewhere, and renew them regularly.

Becoming Left-Handed

WHY DID MY treatment team want me to become left-handed? I kept telling them I'm right-handed, that I was born that way. I write with my right hand. I throw a baseball with my right hand. I kick a soccer ball with my right foot. (I guess I'm right-footed too.) I do everything with my right side. I told them over and over, but they kept saying my life depended on my becoming left-handed.

Slowly I began to attempt to do things using my left side. Writing with my left hand felt awkward and clumsy. Playing sports left-handed felt completely unnatural. In fact, these things felt so bad that I would ultimately give up and go back to using my right side. But everyone kept telling me that feeling awkward, clumsy, and unnatural was normal. These things were actually progress. So eventually I would give being left-handed another shot.

After going through this cycle many times, I can finally say that I'm left-handed. Writing with my left hand and kicking a ball with my left foot actually feels right. I would never even think about going back to using my right side.

Am I serious about becoming left-handed? No. What I am serious about is that fully recovering from my eating disorder felt just like someone had asked me to become left-handed. That would have felt completely wrong. Just like eating the correct amounts of food every day felt completely wrong. Living in my new, healthy body felt incredibly awkward. Dealing with the underlying issues of the eating disorder felt even worse. Learning to have fun, getting enough rest, and letting go of perfectionism felt completely unnatural. To become happy and whole, I had to do all of these things. I essentially became left-handed. And today, as strange as it feels to say, being right-handed—restricting food, being an unhealthy size, being inflexible and rigid, and having no fun—would feel awkward.

Your entire life depends on your becoming left-handed too. For you lefties out there, your lives depend on your becoming right-handed. And for those of you who are ambidextrous—well, you get my point.

The Next Right Thing

I F YOU HAVE read *Life Without Ed*, you might be feeling a little déjà vu right now. Yes, there is a section in my first book called "The Next Right Thing." Don't worry, I'm not duplicating that one. I'm reminding you about an important idea and adding a new twist. I'm actually adding a hubcap. Just wait and see.

The concept of doing the next right thing was critical in my recovery from my eating disorder. If I relapsed, I learned that I needed to get back on track now, not later. After I binged, what I wanted to do was give myself a "break" from food for a while. (Translation: I wanted to stay stuck in my relapse.) What I needed to do was eat the very next meal—no excuses. That's doing the next right thing.

Today this concept is critical in all areas of my life. In relationships, I try to do the next right thing. In my work, I try to do the next right thing. As a citizen of the world, I try to do the next right thing.

Those of us who are in recovery can be grateful that what we have learned, and might not have otherwise, can be used throughout our lives. In Twelve Step meetings, I have often heard people say, "Our past is our greatest asset." Our yesterdays make us better people today.

My friend Rich, who is recovered from alcohol and drug addiction, is just one example of this. As he was driving, he saw a hubcap fall off the car in front of him. The man driving the now-three-hubcapped car didn't notice and kept driving to his destination, which turned out to be Wal-Mart. Without thinking twice, Rich pulled off the road, picked up the hubcap, followed the man to the busy Wal-Mart parking lot, and returned it to him. The man was ecstatic and thanked Rich profusely.

I happened to talk with Rich on the phone right after all this happened. After hearing the story, I said, "Wow! That was really nice of you."

Rich said, "It's no big deal. I'm just doing the next right thing."

My message to you: Pick up the hubcap. Do the next right thing.

Important note: I'm not telling you to follow strangers around in your car, returning things they might lose. What I am saying is carry what you learn in recovery into your life.

Ed-Busters

ARE YOU AN Ed-buster? Maybe you're still struggling with Ed and working hard to kick him out of your life for good. Or maybe you're fully recovered and the divorce is final. Many of you are friends or family members. You don't really understand Ed, but you still fight him on behalf of your loved one. Maybe you're a professional who busts Ed on a regular basis. If you don't consider yourself an Ed-buster, think again. Just by picking up this book, you are learning about eating disorders and aiding in the fight.

As an Ed-buster myself, I hear daily from people who have been touched by an eating disorder and want to work in the eating disorder field. I think it is wonderful that these individuals—many of whom were previously afraid to talk about the illness to anyone—broke through the shame and now want to use their experience to benefit others. I hear from people who want to become therapists, dietitians, doctors, or researchers. Others want to start nonprofit organizations, open treatment centers, or write books and speak about recovery.

Some people who are recovered feel called to work in the eating disorder field. Others don't have this calling, and after recovering, they actually want to get as far away from eating disorders as they possibly can. This might surprise you, but I can actually relate to both experiences.

I felt passionately called to write *Life Without Ed* and *Good-Bye Ed, Hello Me*. Writing and speaking about my recovery has helped me heal. If you can't tell by now, I tend to write and talk about the things I most need to learn. I'm very grateful for the work I've been able to do.

I'm often asked, "How did you begin to share your story?" The funny part is, I couldn't share my story until I had a story to share—and couldn't get that until I focused on my own recovery first. We can't give away what we don't have. Years ago, the women who helped me the most in my therapy group were the ones who were working a solid recovery program themselves. Sure, the other women who weren't doing so well also helped by doing practical things like answering my phone calls and even sitting with me at mealtimes. But absolutely nothing helped me more than the women who actually ate with me. They laughed, smiled, and seemed to be at peace, and that's what I desperately wanted. They gave me hope by example, and in this way, they really didn't have to do anything at all.

Before deciding to speak publicly about your recovery, I highly encourage you to talk with your treatment team about it. Talk about what that would mean in your life. Sharing my story has been a way for me to connect with a core passion I have always had to help others. (That is why I had wanted to go to medical school.) I did not decide to share my story as a way for me to stay connected with the eating disorder identity. In fact, the work that I have done in the eating disorder field has ultimately catapulted me further away from Ed. I know many people for whom this is true, but it is not the case for everyone. For some people, dealing with eating disorders on a regular basis keeps them tied to the illness in an unhealthy way. You must get in touch with your heart and discover what holds true for you.

Instead of remaining involved with eating disorders through work, many people prefer to do something entirely different with their lives, such as becoming teachers, graphic designers, or stay-at-home moms or dads. They prefer to be an example to the world by simply living a healthy lifestyle. In this way, they inspire everyone around them without ever having to mention Ed's name. Some might decide to share their recovery story selectively with people in their lives who they feel might benefit from it. And others might want to make eating disorders a charitable cause for which they volunteer time and energy. We could definitely use more volunteers in this. Imagine if National Eating Disorders Awareness Week, which is sponsored each February by the National Eating Disorders Association (NEDA), could become as large as National Breast Cancer Awareness Month! We just need more involvement to make that happen. (Technically speaking, I suppose we would need a few more weeks too.)

Making eating disorders a part of my work has been frustrating at times. I don't like the fact that sometimes people only think of me as "the woman who recovered from an eating disorder." The truth is I don't want my identity to be based on being *recovered* from an eating disorder any more than I want it to be based on *having* an eating disorder. I want people to know who I really am. As I have said many times in this book, I don't want to give Ed a place in my life. Right now, I work in the eating disorder field, but Ed doesn't have a place in my personal life. He doesn't have anything to do with what I wear, what I eat, who I hang out with, or what I do for fun. Absolutely none. He does, however, have a role in my professional life—I educate other people about him. And that's where things stand today. In the future, this balance for me might shift: I might decide to go back to school and study quantum physics (fascinating stuff) or even try out for *American Idol*. I don't know what the future holds for me, but I do know that it can hold anything at all because I'm recovered.

The same thing goes for you. After you recover, you can do anything. Whether or not you decide to share your story is a personal choice. Like me, you might be surprised that your feelings about this fluctuate. I love the slogan that people who have battled cancer use: "I have cancer, but it doesn't have me." We all may have been touched by an eating disorder, but it doesn't have to define our lives. When we recover, we—as individuals—define our own lives. Don't let Ed take that away from you.

Real Action: Ed-Bustin'

Do you want to take some Ed-bustin' action by helping others? To find the honest answer to this question, go inside yourself and talk with your treatment team. If you are not yet ready, keep bustin' Ed in your own life, and use any desire you may have to help others as motivation to recover fully. If you're interested and ready, visit the Resources section in the back of this book and get involved in organizations that need your support. You could even volunteer with NEDA during National Eating Disorders Awareness Week. Join my e-mail list at jennischaefer.com to stay posted on Ed-bustin' opportunities.

Do the Impossible

RECOVERING FROM AN eating disorder can't be done. It's impossible. Or at least I used to think so.

I did the impossible. I am fully recovered from an eating disorder. You can do the impossible too.

Throughout history, people have done the impossible. We made it to the moon, didn't we? Flying into outer space used to be considered impossible. Now it's commonplace. A space launch hardly makes the news anymore.

When I was a little kid, I remember thinking that riding a bike without training wheels was impossible. Guess what? No training wheels for me.

As a student at Texas A&M University, I thought it would be impossible for me to be a part of the school's vocal jazz octet, the Reveliers, but I sang with them for four years. Not impossible. When I moved to Nashville after college, I thought it would be impossible for me to learn how to play the guitar. I can play a few songs today. I have done the impossible more times than I can count. My guess is that you have too.

Impossible is often just an idea constructed in our minds. As long as we believe something is impossible, it will be. We are bound to ideas produced by our imagination, as demonstrated by one of my favorite stories:

When a baby elephant is tied to a small tree with a rope, it is not strong enough to break free. After trying to break loose repeatedly and failing, the baby elephant will ultimately give up. Years later, the same elephant will not even try to break free if tied to a small tree—despite the fact that an adult elephant could easily uproot even a large tree. As a baby elephant, breaking free was impossible. As an adult elephant, it's quite possible.

Don't be like the elephant. Don't let the past dictate your present.

Maybe you have been in treatment for your eating disorder many times. Maybe you have relapsed over and over. Or maybe you have a marginal recovery and don't think you will ever be really free. It doesn't matter that these things were true for you two years ago, two weeks ago, or two days ago (even two hours ago). That was then. This is now.

Maybe you weren't strong enough then. Maybe you are now. What was once impossible might very well be possible today.

Do the impossible.

Keep Standing

"Fall down seven times, stand up eight." If you have ever attended one of my presentations, read one of my *Ed-buster* newsletters, or visited my MySpace or Facebook pages, you know this Japanese proverb. I use it a lot, because I fell down a lot in my fight for freedom from Ed. In my life after Ed, I kept falling in regard to life stuff. I'm living an amazing life today, not because I never fall, but because I keep standing back up every time I hit the ground. I promise that I have fallen a lot more than seven times, so I have stood up many more than eight times.

If we keep standing, it doesn't matter how many times Ed or life knocks us down, and it doesn't matter how far we fall each time. All that matters is that we keep getting up. Setbacks only become permanent failures when we quit trying. When we feel like giving up, like we are beyond help, we must remember that we are never beyond hope. Holding on to hope has always motivated me to keep trying.

I have often found this hope by connecting with others. I've found it not only in individuals who have dealt with eating disorders but also in people who have battled addictions and those who have survived abuse, cancer, and broken hearts. I have found much-needed hope in my passions and dreams for the future. I've found it in prayer.

Real hope combined with real action has always pulled me through difficult times.

Real hope combined with doing nothing has never pulled me through. In other words, sitting around and simply hoping that things will change won't pick you up after a fall. Hope only gives you strength when you use it as a tool to move forward. Taking real action with a hopeful mind will pull you off the ground that eighth time and beyond.

For those of you who are wondering (because people have asked) how you can stand up eight times if you've only fallen seven, consider this: you began laying flat on the ground.

No matter where you started or how much you fall, just keep standing up—however many times that is!

Real Action: What Works

We all fall in recovery. We all have to find ways to help us fall less along recovery road. One of the most helpful tools for me to avoid relapse was simply making a list called "What Works." I wrote down strategies and tips that had proven reliable in the past to prevent relapse. These were not things that I *thought* worked, but things that I *knew* worked. Over the years, I had many different lists. Here are a few examples taken from one:

1. Call someone and meet face-to-face. Don't just talk on the phone.
2. Commit to writing about your feelings in your journal before bingeing. (If you do this, you might decide not to binge after all.)
3. Move energy in your body by humming deep in your chest. Feel the vibrations.

Make a "What Works" list of your own. Remember to include only things that have been effective in the past.

I kept my list in the back of my journal, because I would continually add to it as I was writing my regular entries. Keep your list in a place where you will see it often. When you're struggling, look at your list and avoid relapse. If you still fall, you know what to do—stand up again!

Don't Have a Backup Plan

I DIDN'T HAVE A backup plan. I was determined to recover from my eating disorder. Sure, in my attempts to fight Ed, I sometimes felt helpless. But as Bill Doyle—my colleague and the father of a young woman recovering from an eating disorder—says, "Don't confuse helplessness with hopelessness." I always had hope, and in the end, I wouldn't settle for anything less than a full recovery.

If you want to make your divorce from Ed final and get on with your life, don't have a backup plan. Don't give yourself a way out. Commit 100 percent to a complete recovery. Do not settle for some mediocre version of recovery.

One of these versions entails living a fairly functional life with the exception of lingering Ed behaviors like avoiding mirrors, dreading restaurants, and counting calories. Don't settle for "fairly functional" and lingering Ed behaviors. Another type of mediocre recovery involves having no problem at all with mirrors, restaurants, or calories, but just being absolutely miserable all the time. I know many more versions because I've lived them. Trust me when I say that there is more out there than mediocre. Go past it to fully recovered and find true joy in an Ed-free life.

Follow one plan: do whatever it takes to make it. Whatever it takes is different for everyone. Find your way. Find people who will support you on your journey.

As you go, don't forget about your dreams and passions. Ed won't forget; he'll try to take them from you. Don't let him. And when it comes to your dreams, don't have a backup plan either. Create your own life. Create your own job. What a strange and exciting concept!

When I decided to write *Life Without Ed*, I didn't have a plan for what I would do if I couldn't find a publisher. I was determined to keep working until I found one who was interested in the book. I didn't know if that would take two months, two years, two decades, or two centuries, but I was in it for the long haul. (If it had taken two centuries, I just wouldn't have been around to experience it.) The point is that I didn't have a fallback. Sometimes I felt helpless, but I always had hope. After recovering from Ed and experiencing that intense level of helplessness, getting a book published was easy. I channeled the energy I had previously put into my eating disorder into writing and other goals. (As you know, that was a lot of energy.) I surrounded myself with people who believed in me and lifted me up.

If you want to be a writer, write; an actor, act; or a banker, bank. I love Henry Ford's quote: "Whether you think that you can, or that you can't, you are usually right." So think you can. With recovery, anything is possible. Gather the tools necessary to pursue your life goals. Maybe you need to go to the library, do research on the Internet, or attend a workshop. Maybe you aspire to be a better mom or dad, sister or brother. Then put energy into that. Connect with supportive people who empower you. The more you jump into your life, the further away from Ed you can get. Don't have a backup plan for living. Live today.

I admit that backup plans are helpful for some things. When it rains at an outdoor wedding, a backup plan keeps the guests dry. For your inner marriage with body, mind, and soul, however, you won't need a backup plan for bad weather. Learn to dance in the rain, and invite others to join you.

Trust in God. Believe in yourself. Get friends and family members to stand behind you. That's the only backup you'll need.

Now go and do it! Go!

"It's Okay to Be Happy"

When I lose ten pounds
And then lose five more
When I'm finally size six
Better yet size four
When I grow my hair
To where it should be
When I look in the mirror
And like what I see
Maybe then maybe then maybe then I'll be happy

When I buy a big house
And I'm out of debt
When I get that job
Have a safety net
When I fall in love
With that perfect guy
I can take a deep breath
I can start my life
Maybe then maybe then maybe then I'll be happy

CHORUS:

That's what I believed that's how I lived
Waiting waiting waiting for that or for this
It was never enough to be where I was
Just enjoying the ride being all right
Knowing whatever life throws at me
It's okay it's okay it's okay to be happy

Don't know when it changed
But somehow it did
Guess I got a little tired
Of the emptiness
So I took some trust
And I got some faith
And when they found each other
I found this place
Where it's okay to be happy

CHORUS:

Now that's what I believe that's how I live
I ain't waiting waiting waiting for that or for this
It was never enough to be where I was
Just enjoying the ride being all right
Knowing whatever life throws at me
It's okay it's okay it's okay to be happy
It's okay it's okay it's okay . . .

BRIDGE:

To be happy
Instead of waiting for the sky to fall
It's okay to be laughing
At the craziness of it all

CHORUS:

Now that's what I believe that's how I live
I ain't waiting waiting waiting for that or for this
I'm just doing my best in this beautiful mess
Just enjoying the ride being all right
Knowing whatever life throws at me
I'll take whatever life throws at me
It's okay it's okay it's okay to be happy

To hear music from Jenni, Dave, and Georgia, visit myspace.com/jennischaefer, myspace.com/davebergmusic, and myspace.com/georgiamiddleman.

Resources

THE FOLLOWING LIST includes only a small sample of what is available. For further resources, visit jennischaefer.com.

Brief descriptions below highlight unique aspects of each organization. Visit websites for additional information.

Organizations

Academy for Eating Disorders (AED)
aedweb.org
847-498-4274
Global professional association for eating disorders research, education, treatment, and prevention

Beating Eating Disorders (BEAT)
www.b-eat.co.uk
Help line: 0845 634 1414; youth line: 0845 634 7650
Charity in the United Kingdom for people with eating disorders and their families

Binge Eating Disorder Association (BEDA)
bedaonline.com
National organization focusing on the need to prevent, diagnose, and treat binge eating disorder

Eating Disorders Anonymous (EDA)
eatingdisordersanonymous.org
Information about free twelve-step meetings focused on balance, not abstinence

Eating Disorders Coalition (EDC)
eatingdisorderscoalition.org
202-543-9570
Advances the federal recognition of eating disorders as a
public health priority through lobby days and other activities

Gürze Books
bulimia.com
800-756-7533
"Eatng Disorders Recovery Today" newletter, books, and
additional resources

**International Association of Eating Disorders Professionals
(iaedp)**
iaedp.com
800-800-8126
Education, training, and certification for eating disorders
professionals

**National Association of Anorexia Nervosa and Associated
Disorders (ANAD)**
anad.org
847-831-3438
Sponsors free support groups worldwide

National Eating Disorders Association (NEDA)
myneda.org
Help line: 800-931-2237
Sponsors National Eating Disorders Awareness Week each
February

National Eating Disorder Information Centre (NEDIC)
nedic.ca
866-633-4220
Canadian site providing information on eating disorders and
weight preoccupation

Websites Related to Jenni's Work

Main website
jennischaefer.com
Mailing list where you can stay posted on speaking
engagements and more

Ed Jewelry
sarah-kate.com
Jewelry designed to raise awareness about eating disorders

Eating Disorders Blogs
eatingdisordersblogs.com
Blog site by Gürze Books (also bulimia.com) addressing
anorexia, bulimia, and other disorders

huffingtonpost.com/jenni-schaefer
Jenni's "Hello Me" blog on *The Huffington Post*

Also be sure to visit Jenni on MySpace.com, Facebook.com, and
Twitter.com.